Practicing Psychology in Rural Settings

Hospital Privileges and Collaborative Care

Edited by

Jerry A. Morris, PsyD

American Psychological Association

Washington, DC

Published by the
American Psychological Association
750 First Street, NE
Washington, DC 20002

Copies may be ordered from
APA Order Department
P.O. Box 92984
Washington, DC 20090-2984

In the United Kingdom and Europe, copies may be ordered from
American Psychological Association
3 Henrietta Street
Covent Garden, London
WC2E 8LU England

Typeset in Palatino by EPS Group Inc., Easton, MD

Printer: Capital City Press, Montpelier, VT
Cover designer: Minker Design, Bethesda, MD
Technical / Production editor: Tanya Y. Alexander

Library of Congress Cataloging-in-Publication Data
Practicing psychology in rural settings : hospital privileges and collaborative care / edited by Jerry A. Morris.
    p.   cm.
  ISBN 1-55798-452-2 (pbk.)
   1. Clinical psychology—Practice—United States. 2. Rural mental health services—United States. 3. Hospitals—United States—Medical staff—Clinical privileges. I. Morris, Jerry A.
  RC467.95.P7 1997
  362.2'0425—dc21

                         97-25216
                           CIP

British Library Cataloguing-in-Publication Data
A CIP record is available from the British Library.

Printed in the United States of America
First edition

Contents

Contributors

James H. Bray, *Baylor College of Medicine, Houston, TX*

Paul L. Craig, *Anchorage, AK*

Michael F. Enright, *Jackson, WY*

David S. Hargrove, *University of Mississippi, University, MS*

James G. Hill, *American Psychological Association, Office of Rural Health, Washington, DC*

Peter A. Keller, *Mansfield University, Mansfield, PA*

Mary Beth Kenkel, *California School of Professional Psychology, Fresno*

Sue A. Kuba, *California School of Professional Psychology, Fresno*

Jerry A. Morris, *Community Mental Health Consultants, Inc., Nevada, MO*

Robert J. Resnick, *Virginia Commonwealth University, Richmond*

John Rogers, *Baylor College of Medicine, Houston, TX*

Ronald H. Rozensky, *The Evanston Hospital, Evanston, IL*

Foreword

Psychologists in rural areas stand in the forefront of a movement in American psychology to obtain hospital privileges and practice collaboratively in primary care settings. Practicing psychologists have long recognized the importance of continuity of care for their patients. This continuity can be maintained through collaborative practice with primary care physicians, but is often interrupted when psychologists' patients must be hospitalized. Only a few states and jurisdictions (17) have passed laws authorizing psychologists to practice in a hospital setting. Doctors of psychology have been frustrated and angered by the failure of the hospital system to recognize the depth and breadth of their training and the need for continuity of care for psychologists' patients. Furthermore, once patients are hospitalized, they are often misunderstood and their psychological needs are poorly integrated into an inpatient medical system. Without mechanisms to support psychological leadership and intervention, the patients' psychological problems are not treated and both their long-term psychological and physical health are compromised.

Rural psychologists are taking the lead in protecting the quality of their patients' behavioral health care. Rural settings are, perforce, more conducive to interdisciplinary and collaborative practice due to the scarcity of health providers in general. Rural states are, therefore, more likely to pass authorizing legislation for psychologists' hospital privileges. By expanding the scope of psychologists' practice to include hospitals, states can ensure the continuity of behavioral health care for rural residents.

State by state, psychologists are attaining hospital privileges and will become able to serve their patients more effectively. In addition, it is expected that psychologists will expand their collaboration with primary care physicians to meet the behavioral health needs of rural patients. Often, the teamwork between a psychologist and a family physician offers the most comprehensive behavioral and physical health services. But with this expansion of scope of practice comes the need to prepare psychologists for these new roles in hospital and primary care environments.

In response to that need, the Committee on Rural Health of the American Psychological Association has developed this volume. Although its focus is on primary care practice in rural areas, the principles of practice can be applied to other areas as well. Practitioners everywhere would be wise to avail themselves of this manual and prepare themselves for the eventuality of primary care and hospital practice in their states.

Dorothy Cantor, PsyD

Preface

This volume is designed to aid the rural psychologist in educating hospital board members, medical staff members as well as chiefs of medical services, and rural citizens about some of the contributions rural psychologists make in hospital settings. It has some usefulness as a brief and introductory instrument in educating and recruiting the rural psychologist to the hospital setting, increasing psychologists' awareness of the psychological and related physical health issues that may be emphasized in early discussions with hospital staff and administrators as pertinent to the development of psychological services. The volume may be useful as a general overview and reading supplement in the training of psychologists who may practice in the rural community or who venture into sparsely populated areas as a part of their consulting practice.

The volume is therefore introductory and does not pretend to survey all the contributions psychologists make in the rural hospital. Rural contributions to general behavioral and physical health, trauma rehabilitation, oncology services, cardiac rehabilitation, pediatric programs, and so forth are omitted due to the limitations associated with this publication. Certainly there are a wealth of collaborative opportunities and special populations that are not covered in this book for the sake of brevity.

This work represents a model of what collaboration can accomplish. A special vote of thanks goes to the American Psychological Association (APA) Board of Directors for their firm and constant support for rural and frontier psychologists, and for their advocacy for rural patient access to psychological services. The Board was resoundingly joined by the APA Council of Representatives, which provided funding for this project, and the Women's Work Group of the APA Rural Health Task Force.

Working with James Barron, PhD, who took this project as consulting editor with the ensuing short deadlines and hard work out of a commitment to psychology and personal friendship, has been a joy. Dr. Barron's talents, work ethic, and willingness to fit this very important project into a very busy schedule solidified the final product. His family is to be commended for loaning Jim to us.

The APA Rural Health Task Force has honed itself into a talented, energetic, and task-oriented group of professionals interested in improving rural psychology training, services, research, and practice opportunities. Importantly, these task force members who have become great friends are hard working, generous, and welcoming of diversity. The task force members contributed the bulk of the chapters in this volume.

The Hospital and Health Care Committee of APA's Division of Independent Practice (Division 42) has a long tradition of publication, advocacy for hospital psychologists, and interest in the rural and community hospital. The committee contributed three members who added chapters, assisted with costs, and were outstandingly dependable and committed to advocacy for the hospital practice of psychology in rural settings.

Most important, the rock upon which we built this project was my administrative assistant, Candi Dahmer. Her unwavering flexibility and ability to fit this project into our overwhelming calendar of commitments and deadlines were no less than miraculous. Every author got to know and appreciate Candi, and called on her extensive talents.

Finally, a great reverence and vote of appreciation must be raised for those rural physicians, hospital administrators and board members, and psychologists who have courageously established hospital psychological services for patients. These pioneers have contributed greatly to the quality of care in the American rural hospital. Rural hospital leadership (administrators, chiefs of medical service, and board members) seeking to develop or refine hospital psychological services may receive information, technical assistance, and referral to state psychological associations by contacting the APA's Office of Rural Health, The Division of Independent Practice (Division 42; see the Appendix), or by calling state psychological associations.

Jerry A. Morris, PsyD
Editor

Acknowledgments

The Rural Health Task Force of the American Psychological Association (APA) is committed to enhancing the psychological and behavioral health of people living in rural and frontier America. To this end, the task force has been working since 1991 to open communications with traditional health care providers and health service delivery systems in isolated and underserved communities.

Because of its successes, the task force was elevated to the permanent status of a formal and ongoing committee of the APA in 1996. This volume was prepared with special resources set aside by the APA Council of Representatives to facilitate a better understanding of the wide variety of roles psychologists play in rural hospitals and health facilities. This publication was also supported by the Hospital and Health Care Facilities Committee of the APA Division of Psychologists in Independent Practice (Division 42). Jerry Morris, PsyD, chairs this committee and is also a member of the Rural Health Task Force. Gratitude is extended to Dr. Morris, who worked as the primary author of this volume.

Further thanks are extended to James G. Hill, director of APA's Office of Rural Health, for coordinating the production of this volume and to James Barron, PhD, for participating with Dr. Morris in editing the final draft. Finally, the members of the Rural Health Task Force—James Bray, PhD; Sylvia Shellenberger, PhD; Mary Beth Kenkel, PhD; Paul Craig, PhD; and Arthur McDonald, PhD—are acknowledged for their contributions, support, technical assistance, and overwhelming good fellowship in producing this publication.

Michael F. Enright, PhD, ABPP
Chair
APA Rural Health Task Force 1993–1996

Introduction: Background and Context

James W. Barron

A biomedical philosophy has prevented the full and independent practice of psychology in hospital settings. The excitement and contributions of the golden era of biological and medical science, coupled with the development of sometimes dangerous biological interventions, resulted in the tradition of close restriction of hospital practice to the physician. Psychologists' participation as admitting and attending doctors in hospitals was delayed by the displacement of the very real fear of the potential side effects of medical misdiagnosis and interventions to all doctors regardless of their training and discipline.

Consequently, the nonphysician practitioner wishing to hospitalize his or her patient to gain strict control of the patient's practices and environment, and to foster the linkage of comprehensive and coordinated multidisciplinary care, was viewed as biologically endangering. It was assumed that concern for the patient's welfare, the intelligence and training required to link the patient with appropriate services and specialists, and decisiveness and capacity to ensure the patient's safety were embodied in foundational biophysiological training.

Over time, clinically trained psychologists began to be well enough disbursed to provide administrators, board members, patients, and the public with firsthand examples of the effectiveness of psychological interventions and leadership. The public's awareness of and demand for the services of psychologists accelerated the growth of opportunities in rural and frontier communities where doctors of all varieties were in short supply. Psychologists found the rural community open and flexible, delighted to attract all variety of doctors. As a result, psychologists became cognizant of the opportunities to practice and to make meaningful contributions in rural hospital environments, and often established successful, well-respected practices.

Activists within the American Psychological Association (APA) established an organizational priority of advancing psychologists' practice in hospital settings. They created supportive structures, mobilized resources, and spearheaded efforts to bring about necessary legal and regulatory changes to enable psychologists to make full use of their training in inpatient settings. Rural hospital administrators and medical directors, desiring to strengthen clinical services and to compete more effectively in the health care marketplace, began to include psychologists on multidisciplinary teams.

Ultimately, the demand for a broad scope of psychological practice and leadership grew out of an increasing public awareness of the effects of personality, lifestyle, and habit on long-term health and disease control, and appreciation for the limitations of a strict biological approach to disease. This public interest in psychological approaches to treatment and prevention, the emergence of economic trends that encouraged institutions to broaden their support of psychological doctors, and the proven effectiveness of many psychological assessment and intervention techniques resulted in the evolution of regulations and laws relating to hospital practice, and the opportunity for hospitals to develop more comprehensive staffing and programs that include psychological treatments.

This volume provides the rural psychologist, hospital administration and board, and medical staff with a general introduction to the history and parameters of the development of the conditions that facilitate the participation of doctors of psychology in hospital programs. The foundations for establishing a hospital practice, the components of collaboration between psychologists and medical staff that will ultimately strengthen the quality of hospital programs and the breadth of patient choice are discussed. Examples of several of the specific populations that benefit from the inclusion of psychologists on hospital staffs and in program leadership are provided.

This book is the initial tool for rural hospital psychologists to use for brief background information and ultimately the establishment of a common set of ideas, information, and issues for discussion to initiate meetings and planning for the implementation or expansion of psychology privileges in hospitals. Although the contributions of the psychologist in the hospital are by no means covered in depth and expansively in this volume, the reader will achieve a basic understanding of the road psychologists have traveled to establish patient access to psychology-related health solutions and leadership in hospitals. The reader is provided with examples of ways psychologists in many rural hospitals are improving patient care; contributing to the survival of the facilities; and learning the commitments, processes, and responsibilities attendant to hospital practice.

Recommendations for the Future

The rural delivery system of the future must be centered around the primary care clinic and community hospital. This model is the only one that can provide access, early intervention, coordination, and collaboration, and overcome the fragmentation, recruiting difficulties, and cost problems of rural delivery systems. Rural psychologists should urge governmental agencies and rural hospitals to adopt the following principles to provide access, early intervention, and coordination:

1. Mental health problems occur in high prevalence in the general population, and therefore a broadened definition of primary health care that includes mental health practitioners working in conjunction with generalist physicians at the rural hospital and primary health care center must be developed.

2. Because many physical health problems have a significant cognitive and behavioral component, a balanced approach using a multidisciplinary team is indicated in the rural hospital and primary care delivery system. Such multidisciplinary systems should undergo cost and outcome ef-

fectiveness testing against the traditional physician and nurse intervention model.

3. The current system must be modified to provide the consumer of health care services with a broad array of practitioner, modality, and cost choices relative to the diagnosis, prevention, and amelioration of physical health, substance abuse, and mental health problems. This modification is particularly important at the rural hospital, which is the only viable resource in many rural communities for maintaining psychological specialists.

4. Managed care (health maintenance and preferred provider organizations and Medicaid and Medicare types of coordinated benefit systems) and rural hospitals should give financial incentives for rural psychology hospital and primary care practice development. These incentives should encourage expansion that offers comprehensive diagnosis and treatment planning by a physician, psychologist, or both; multidisciplinary team treatment systems; implementation of strong behavioral prevention and case-management programs; and use of balanced biological and behavioral approaches. To qualify for the incentives, a program should ensure that the systems are comprehensive, involve local rather than regional service delivery and accessibility, make holistic programs available, and can demonstrate cost and utilization effectiveness.

5. Rural hospitals should establish recruitment efforts to hire psychologists with the skills necessary to provide behavioral health models of practice in the hospital and local outpatient primary care setting. These hospitals should use their financial and leadership leverage to collaborate with primary care centers to position these psychology doctors prominently in their outpatient and inpatient programs.

Organization of This Volume

Part I of this volume explores the foundations of establishing a hospital practice. The discipline of rural psychology has matured over the past 30 years. The number of psychologists providing an array of essential clinical services in rural hospital environments has grown steadily. Resnick and Morris describe in chapter 1 rural psychology's roots in the strategies and values of community psychology: recognition of social and environmental factors in changing behaviors; utilization of systems-oriented interventions; identification and treatment of targeted populations; emphasis on prevention; mobilization and management of community resources; active outreach; development of innovative programs; and close collaboration with other professionals in the health care delivery systems.

To aid both psychologists and health care executives in their analyses of issues of professional medical staff membership, responsibilities, and privileges, Rozensky summarizes (chapter 2) relevant history and current practice. Since 1985, regulations of the Joint Commission on Accreditation of Health Care Organizations (JCAHO) have authorized the inclusion of nonphysicians on medical staffs. Rozensky explores the complex intersection of membership issues with professional licensing; JCAHO regulations; state and federal laws; Medicare, Medicaid, and other insurance reimbursements; freedom of choice; consumer satisfaction; and, most important, standards, ethics, and quality of care.

In chapter 3, Morris explains how the transition to organized systems of care based on a restricted understanding of "medical necessity" and a strong preference for outpatient services has resulted in major changes in the hospital industry. As managed health care principles become more influential on hospital policy, cost containment and profits emerge as priorities for hospitals rather than a strict patient-oriented philosophy of care. The hospital psychologist is uniquely trained and positioned to fill the emerging need for rapid mental health and behavioral interventions followed by competent outpatient care, allowing the hospital increased opportunity to transition patient care.

Part II of this volume focuses on collaboration and linkages with other health care professionals. In chapter 4, Bray, Enright, and Rogers take a careful look at the differences in "culture," education, training, methods, goals, and practice styles of physicians and psychologists. The authors make a strong case for analyzing those differences so that they do not become insurmountable obstacles and genuine collaboration can occur.

No single health care discipline or program can meet the complex, diverse physical and mental health needs of patients in rural settings. Various disciplines and programs comprise subsystems that must link to form an integrated whole. Hargrove and Keller (chapter 5) explore the importance of interdisciplinary communication, cooperation, and collaboration with community mental health centers that provide a broad range of inpatient, outpatient, and rehabilitation services. They emphasize the need for conceptualized models of collaboration, although much work remains to be done in this area. Psychologists need to participate in developing and implementing a variety of models that can foster mutually respectful reciprocal interdisciplinary relationships.

Psychologists work in many different domains within the rural hospital environment, but their services in the rural hospital emergency room may be the most critical. As Morris emphasizes, medical emergencies frequently have significant behavioral and psychological components that require psychologists' knowledge-base, assessment, consultation, crisis intervention, and treatment skills to respond fully to the needs of patients and their families. Morris concludes that the psychologist and physician make an especially powerful combination in the rural health care environment.

Finally, Part III of this volume provides examples of how psychological treatment can aid special populations in hospital practice. Rural health care administrators and providers are working to identify the needs of special populations and to develop responsive programs and services. Craig, in chapter 7, demonstrates that the discipline of clinical neuropsychology is integral to the diagnosis, treatment, and rehabilitation of such patients. Neuropsychologists, with their unique theoretical and methodological base, work collaboratively with primary care physicians, neurologists, and other specialists, significantly improving the quality of care rendered to brain-injured patients.

In chapter 8, Kuba and Kenkel describe the innovative approaches to meeting the needs of women, particularly in the area of overlapping boundaries where physical and psychological health care interact. These integrative approaches emphasize prevention, early diagnosis, active outreach, and a variety of psychoeducational programs addressing the special concerns of women. Kuba and Kenkel assert that careful attention to women's health care, in addition to benefiting women directly, has a salutary effect on the entire organized system of health care, helping administrators and providers to become more aware of the multifaceted, biopsychosocial elements that interact to cause illness and that, if understood properly, can contribute to health.

From a similar vantage point, Morris and Hill (chapter 9) view the treatment of patients with alcohol and other substance abuse and addiction problems. These services require multidisciplinary teams made up of substance abuse counselors and educators, case managers, nurses, primary care physicians, and psychologists. Morris and Hill describe the important roles psychologists play in the delivery, coordination, and management of these services at the hospital and in outpatient settings.

Conclusion

Despite the richness of these examples, they can only be illustrative of the important, diverse roles psychologists play in health care systems in rural environments. As an educative tool, this volume highlights the contributions of psychologists' knowledge of human behavior and related clinical skills to the solutions of wide-ranging physical and behavioral health care problems.

Rural psychology is no longer new but it remains a pioneering field. The models of cooperation, consultation, interdisciplinary teamwork, innovative program development, and integration of services have potential applicability and usefulness to the entire system of health care in this country. Initiatives to fully deploy rural psychologists in the hospital and primary care system will facilitate improved quality of care, cost–benefit interplay, and consumer choice in the emerging health care system. Visionary hospital administrators, boards, chiefs of medical staff, and psychologists need to advocate for broadened psychologist involvement in the rural hospital.

I

Foundations of Establishing a Hospital Practice

1

The History of Rural
Hospital Psychology

Robert J. Resnick and Jerry A. Morris

The rural city, county, or regional hospital is the heart of the health care delivery system. It is the place where scarce professional resources come together. The rural patient perceives the hospital as a safety net, a vital bulwark against disaster, calamity, and even death. As an institution it represents a part of local inhabitants' history and tradition rather than simply "a choice of hospitals." The rural hospital is the shared island in which friends and family are born and survive trauma, neighbors are employed, and many individuals say goodbyes to associates and loved ones. The rural hospital is the fishbowl in which the community watches and whispers; in which doctors and staff cooperate or squabble and treat each other with respect or disdain; and in which miracles or tragedies occur.

In the rural community hospital, the health practitioner is frequently a long-term presence. Unlike the urban practitioner who, in conflict, can simply move to the hospital across town, the rural practitioner who is uncomfortable, or unwelcome, at the local hospital often faces uprooting family and practice. The rural specialist, closed out of full participation at the local hospital, is often deprived of access to many patients, is prevented from using many of his or her most useful techniques and skills, and is isolated and alienated professionally.

The rural hospital is therefore an important institution and symbol in the rural community. In this context rural psychologists began to forge an impact during the mid-1960s. These pioneering doctors settled in rural areas for many reasons. Some grew up in rural areas and appreciated the people, environment, and lifestyle. Others sought frontiers where their skills could make a difference. Still others left memories and systems in the urban areas to seek flexible environments. Whatever the reason for practice in the rural setting, the rural psychologist understands the importance of the community hospital in the service delivery network.

Rural Psychology's Roots in Community Psychology

Organized psychology's response to practice in rural settings "officially" dates to the Boston Conference on Community Psychology in 1965 (Bennett, 1965; Bennett et al., 1966; Korchin, 1976). This conference resulted in the American Psychological Association's (APA) establishment of a Division of Community Psychology.

The first community mental health journal, focusing on psychological knowledge related to rural practice, was also founded in 1965 (Korchin, 1976). By 1973, two new journals covering community psychology were launched. Community psychology asserted the importance of social and environmental factors in changing behavior, supported systems-oriented interventions, and advocated prevention and the treatment of targeted populations rather than just the alleviation of psychopathology. The community psychologist focused on the management of local community resources and caretakers as well as the psychological condition of the patient, and actively reached out to patients and groups to foster early identification and intervention. These psychologists adopted ecological approaches with flexible intervention styles and modalities as a vehicle to develop innovative programs. They tapped into whichever resources were available on the local level to solve psychological problems and to foster constructive social reform.

The early community psychologist (and later the subvariant, rural psychologist) embraced the concepts of collaboration, patient advocacy, networking, and team treatment. These concepts became the hallmark of rural practice and meshed nicely with the psychologist's training in the management of group dynamics, the development of behavioral paradigms, and the refinement and objectification of data. Soon rural psychologists who came to "small-town America" with little more than a suitcase, a box of books, and scientific training and practice became valuable members of the rural treatment force, with a significant cadre of patients who depended on them for services.

The rural psychologist began to integrate the principles of psychological science and practice with the often sparsely available grassroots agencies and resources. These included the clergy and religious institutions, social service agencies, law enforcement, the courts, school districts, state mental health authorities, primary care physicians, and the community hospital.

Generally, most patients are treated by primary care providers in primary care institutions (Brody, 1996; Regier, Goldberg, & Taube, 1978; Schulberg & Scott, 1991). The rural psychologist, trained to treat both psychological problems and the behavioral aspects of physical disease, had to follow patients into primary care settings (Morris, 1995).

Early Demand for Psychologists' Services

In 1978, California enacted the first hospital privileges act giving statutory permission for hospitals to admit doctors of psychology to medical staffs and to accord them admitting and attending privileges (Enright, Resnick, Ludwigsen, & DeLeon, 1993). In 1978, 5% of medical schools in the United States granted full privileges to psychology faculty members who often treated inpatients and acted as training professors for medical students (Thompson & Matarazzo, 1984). This figure grew rapidly. By 1983, 13% of medical schools in the United States granted full privileges to psychologist faculty members in hospitals (Carr, 1987; Litwin, Boswell, & Kraft, 1991; Thompson, 1987). In 1982, 10% of all psychologists were working primarily in hospitals (Manderscheid & Sonnenschein, 1991). During the early 1980s, many psychologists began to fill a noteworthy need, becoming independent contractors for hospitals and health care facilities and providing diagnostic and treatment services (Mickel, 1982).

Hospitals became aware of the antitrust implications of excluding psychologists from hospital staffs (Bersoff, 1983). As the demand for psychological services grew, organized efforts to block hospital privileges for psychologists grew among psychiatrists (Fink, 1986), and a decade or more of turf warfare ensued, with the courts ultimately deciding in favor of psychologists.

A major trend toward the privatization of the hospital industry began in the mid-1980s. As the for-profit corporations took over much of the hospital industry, owners and administrators began to assertively demand the right to employ psychologists and to make psychological services available to patients and their families (Gaylin, 1985; Schlesinger & Dorwart, 1984). Psychologists became a recognized force in hospitals and began to request standards and guidance from the APA regarding the practice of psychology in hospitals.

In the fall of 1984, APA and its Board of Professional Affairs (BPA) authorized a task force to write *A Hospital Practice Primer for Psychologists* (APA, 1985). This document ushered in the era of the formalization of a national agenda to make hospital psychological services available to the general public. Later, BPA formed the Task Force on Advocacy for Hospital Practice and the Task Force on Privileging and Credentialing whose recommendations later became official APA policy.

The Growth of Public and Psychologist Awareness of Hospital Psychology

By the mid-1980s psychologists were in hospitals in sufficient numbers to be making noteworthy contributions to patient diagnosis and care. Often, rural hospitals and physicians were willing to include the psychologist because of shortages of psychiatrists, the need for assistance with overwhelming workloads, and the professional isolation. Rural psychologists benefited from these phenomena and seized the opportunity to prove themselves by making meaningful contributions to the rural hospital and to patient care. Soon, awareness of close professional relationships and comfortable collaboration between rural physicians and psychologists began to be expressed in the literature and at professional society meetings (Enright & Blue, 1989).

By 1985, the APA developed a manual describing the role of psychologists in hospitals (APA, 1985). Exposed to the teachings of psychologists–professors holding appointments on medical school faculties and hospital staffs, newly trained physicians acquired greater familiarity with psychological knowledge and skills. The experiences of family physicians who collaborated with psychologists led to the formation of psychologist–physician teams. The stage was set for the formalization of rural psychological hospital practice along collegial and mutually respectful lines.

Legal and Regulatory Changes

By 1984, 44% of psychologists in California indicated that they provided hospital services to patients (Patterns of Psychological Practice Survey, 1984). The number of psychologists practicing in health care settings had increased from 20,126 in 1974 to 45,536 in 1985 (Dorken, Stapp, & VandenBos, 1986). During the mid- to late 1980s major innovation occurred in the area of cost-effective psychological interventions in hospitals and health care settings (Enright et al., 1993). These innovations dramatically increased the demand and use of psychological services in public general hospitals (McCarrick, Rosenstein, Milanzo-Sayre, & Manderscheid, 1988). The psychological and hospital literature began to point out the critical need for psychological approaches in the hospital (Elefant, 1985).

These developments furthered the schism between psychi-

atrists and psychologists as competition for patients intensified. Fink (1986), past president of the American Psychiatric
Association, identified what he deemed a dangerous trend toward psychologists' achieving privileges in hospitals and cited
concern that family physicians and psychologists were collaborating on the treatment of patients with psychological–
behavioral problems. Clearly, the trend in the numbers of psychologists collaborating with physicians in hospitals was
increasing dramatically (Matarazzo, Lubin, & Nathan, 1978;
Zaro, Batchelor, Ginsberg, & Pallak, 1982).

Psychiatry and psychology were at an impasse. Psychiatry's entrenched position was to characterize psychologists
as undertrained and dangerous to patients. The influence of
psychiatrists on indemnity plan boards resulted in some insurers refusing to pay doctors of psychology, echoing psychiatrist's concerns about the adequacy of psychological
training. Earlier, in 1977, psychologists began to take a formal
stand against these characterizations and turf battle issues.
In the precedent-setting Virginia Blues Case (see Resnick,
1985), a psychologist asserted that doctors of psychology
with an average of 7 years of postbaccalaureate training, 1
year of internship, and 1 to 3 years of postdoctoral residency
are adequately trained to diagnose and treat mental illness.
The court determined that psychologists do not represent a
public health hazard as asserted by psychiatry, but that their
presence actually enhances the quality of services to patients
(Resnick, 1985). This public stand by a psychologist and his
supporters established access to psychological services by
giving patients the right to apply their insurance coverage to
the practitioner of their choice.

Another important breakthrough occurred in the mid-
1980s. In 1985, the Joint Commission on Accreditation of
Healthcare Organizations (JCAHO) decided to allow hospitals to include nonphysician providers on professional/med-
ical staffs (Enright, Resnick, Ludwigsen, & DeLeon, 1993).
Since 1985, the JCAHO *Accreditation Manual for Hospitals* has
stated that the organized medical staff includes fully licensed
physicians, and may include other licensed individuals permitted by law and by the hospital, to provide patient care

independently (JCAHO, 1992). In its 1991 accreditation manual, the JCAHO (1991) required a single organized medical staff and specifically recognized licensed nonphysician professionals permitted to practice by state statute.

By this time, changes in the level of competition in the hospital industry made psychologists with hospital privileges and large outpatient practices attractive as contributors to hospital patient census (Dafter & Freeland, 1988; Enright et al., 1993). The advent of increasing indemnity plan coverage, public demand for psychological services, strong support from the national association (APA), and the ability to refer patients to hospitals led to the active recruitment of psychologists for hospital staff membership.

By 1989, 15.7% of psychologists were employed full time in hospitals or medical school settings (APA, Office of Demographic, Employment, and Educational Research, 1989). At the end of the 1980s, psychologists had established a significant presence in nursing homes and were contributing to patient care in those inpatient settings (Bootzin, Shadish, & McSweeny, 1989). During the late 1980s and early 1990s, substantial modifications to the federal statutes governing Medicare gave psychologists autonomous practice permission under the Omnibus Budget Reconciliation Act (1988). Psychologists' increased presence in hospitals and nursing homes, on medical school faculties and teaching hospital staffs, and autonomous functioning in indemnity plans and Medicare brought psychology to a position of credibility and importance in hospitals and health facilities.

The advocacy for patients needing psychological services in hospitals eventually required court intervention and had to be dealt with as a patient right rather than as a discipline or theoretical supremacy issue. As American psychology began its second century, California psychologists challenged the barriers to accessible psychological services in hospital settings. Psychologists fought the legal arguments that only physicians were capable of full hospital admitting and attending privileges. Although psychologists had had statutory admitting and attending privileges since 1978 (Enright et al., 1993), the California court held that the special skills of a physician were needed to admit, attend, and discharge patients in hospitals because of the need to evaluate patients' physical conditions.

Psychologists maintained that their training and expertise prepared them to perform gross screening of medical symptoms and to refer patients for physician evaluation when indicated. They maintained that they were qualified to perform mental diagnosis, write appropriate treatment or consultation orders, act as the attending doctor, and make placement and discharge decisions.

The case went all the way to the California Supreme Court, which held that a psychologist is trained and qualified to act as an admitting and attending doctor in hospital settings (*CAPP v. Rank*, 1990). In fact, by 1991, the American Psychiatric Association Task Force on Medical Staff Bylaws, in the American Medical Association's (1991) Statements on Delineation of Hospital Privileges, indicated that psychiatrists cannot define the training of another discipline and therefore cannot address the training of a nonpsychiatrist practitioner. This publication maintained that the decision about the best way to accomplish quality care in hospitals must be made by each hospital's governing board with due consideration of state and federal law. The *CAPP v. Rank* landmark decision sparked a serious dialogue about the independent and full attending role of psychologists in hospitals (Enright, Resnick, DeLeon, Sciara, & Tanney, 1990).

As hospital practice for psychologists flourished and became increasingly defined by statute, national association literature, and the courts, psychologists began to establish guidelines relative to ethical and malpractice issues arising from inpatient practice (Pope, 1990). Leaders in psychology seriously considered a range of hospital-related issues that were based on maintaining the integrity of the profession and the humane and effective treatment of patients (Mozdzierz, Snodgrass, & DeLeon, 1992). This knowledge base and national leadership converged on the extension of professional psychology in hospitals. In August 1991, the APA Council of Representatives (APA's national legislative and policy-making body) adopted a policy for credentialing psychologists in hospitals and health care facilities (Enright et al., 1993). Subsequently, APA (1991) published the *Guidelines on Hospital Privileges: Credentialing and Bylaws* to establish uniform procedures and standards for establishing and reviewing psychologists' privileges in hospitals.

The establishment of the scope of practice of psychologists in hospital settings had an impact on psychologists' participation in medical schools and teaching hospitals. For example, the number of psychologists employed on U.S. medical school faculties had grown to 3,000 by 1991 (Sweet, Rozensky, & Tovian, 1991). VandenBos, DeLeon, and Belar (1991) reported that 20% of nursing school faculty who were trained at the doctoral level were psychologists. By the early 1990s, psychologists had become important faculty members and trainers for the preparation of hospital practitioners in psychology, medicine, and nursing.

Soon states were rapidly modifying their hospital rules and regulations to allow psychologists expanded practice and admitting and attending privileges in hospitals (Ludwigsen, 1992, 1993). California, Florida, Georgia, Iowa, Louisiana, Maryland, North Carolina, Ohio, Wisconsin, and the District of Columbia were the first to establish statutory authority for psychologist practice (Ludwigsen, 1993; Ludwigsen & Albright, 1994). By October 1993, 11 states and jurisdictions had enacted hospital privileges for psychologists (Cullen, 1993). By 1996, Connecticut, Hawaii, Missouri, New Jersey, New Mexico, Oklahoma, and Utah had been added to this list, with a large group of additional states with legislation pending—for a total of 16 states plus the District of Columbia. In states where there is no permissive legislation or where existing language is silent regarding hospital practice, psychologists provide services by virtue of their state licensure acts granting psychologists diagnostic and treatment authority and defining their scope of practice.

From 1993 to 1995, many psychologists functioned as members of hospital staffs. However, their full autonomy was restricted by a section of the Social Security Act requiring physician supervision of all treatment and of nonphysician professionals in hospitals participating in federal reimbursement (Social Security Administration, 1993). Patients suffering from mental illness and the behavioral correlates of physical illness were increasingly choosing psychologists as their doctors. Many state laws, insurers, and accrediting bodies had long since come to view psychologists as fully autonomous practitioners adequately trained to diagnose and direct the treatment of mental disorders and the behavioral components of physical problems. However, many hospital administrators and medical staffs under pressure of Social Security Act regulation were concerned about losing their Medicaid and Medicare certification if physician supervision was not strictly maintained.

After adverse Health Care Financing Administration (HCFA, 1989) reviews made a chilling impact on psychologists' practices in hospitals, the APA mounted a congressional campaign and HCFA negotiations concerning the loss of patients' access to psychologists' services. HCFA field surveyors were intimidating hospitals with the potential loss of Medicaid and Medicare participation (reimbursement) by issuing negative site visit findings when psychologists functioned as full doctors without (or with limited) supervision. Many of these reviewers had been trained prior to legislative and rule and regulation changes at the federal and state levels and had not integrated new standards into their review practices. The HCFA is generally slow to update training materials and programs and simply circulates bulletins that are easily missed or ignored by site visitors.

Among usually conservative hospital administrators and boards with millions of dollars of revenue at stake, a single uniformed HCFA site visitor in a region can send a chilling effect rippling through hospitals regarding psychological services. The complexity of existing standards, constant and evolving congressional and state changes in regulatory statute and rule, and the fact that most HCFA reviewers are part-time consultants, in one medical specialty, dramatically increase the likelihood of misinterpretation and misinformation during and shortly after HCFA reviews.

In 1995, Congress modified section 1861f of the Social Security Act to allow psychologists to act as autonomous attending doctors primarily responsible for the treatment of patients under their direct care in hospitals and health care facilities (Social Security Administration, 1993). This change removed a major barrier to the enactment of state statutes ensuring that patients have access to psychological services in hospitals and other health care facilities. In rural hospitals, general physicians can now share with fully recognized specialists in psychology the treatment responsibilities for patients with mental illness or serious behavioral problems affecting their physical condition.

In recent years, even the conservative Veterans Administration (VA) has modified its prohibition against psychologists' privileges and membership on medical staffs. In 1994, formal VA policy was modified to grant each VA medical center on a facility-by-facility basis the authority to provide psychologists with medical staff privileges (Enright et al., 1993). Psychologists in many VA hospitals are now making contributions by providing the full range of psychological services and directing patient care with resulting increases in quality of care.

Rural Psychologists' Special Contributions

By the mid-1990s, changes in the health care system were causing psychologists to become affiliated with hospital systems in order to ensure inclusion on managed care panels and contracts (Ludwigsen & Albright, 1994). This trend was especially apparent in rural areas where most managed care organizations view the hospital, and its staff members, as the only essential ingredient in establishing a network. These corporations established initial contact with hospitals and worked through their professional staff to create the foundation of the local health contracting network.

Rural hospital psychologists began to address the problem of medical practitioner diagnostic and screening limitations relative to mentally ill and psychologically encumbered patients. While medical specialists were correctly identifying mental illness in screened patients only 10% to 50% of the time (Nielsen & Williams, 1980; Schulberg, Saul, McClelland, et al., 1985), psychologists joined emergency room staffs and improved these services. Many medical specialists have admitted their training and practice limitations in these areas and have generally welcomed the inclusion of specialists who can improve the quality of care for patients with serious psychological disorders or behavioral problems related to physical illness (Borges, Summers, & Karshmer, 1995).

Psychologists in rural hospitals are making significant contributions to quality, outcome, and cost-effectiveness. Evidence is mounting that the more psychotherapy and related psychological services patients in certain treatment populations receive, the better the outcome (Baker, Jodrey, Intagliatia, & Straus, 1993; Durell, Lechtenberg, Corse, & Frances, 1993; McLellan, Arndt, Metzger, Woody, & O'Brien, 1993). Rural psychologists, therefore, make an economically efficient and therapeutically effective contribution to the health care system. Hospital administrators, physicians, and patients appreciate this contribution and are increasingly including psychologists on hospital staffs (APA, Office of Demographic, Employment, and Educational Research, 1989).

Conclusion

Rural psychologists respond to the delivery system centered around the rural hospital and related agencies and to the growing economic incentives to affiliate with the hospital. Decreasing regulatory and statutory barriers to psychological practice in hospitals caused rural psychologists to actively seek hospital privileges. These psychologists bring to rural hospitals experience in the diagnosis and treatment of mental illness and psychological distress. Collaboration with physicians on the behavioral and psychosocial aspects of physical illness have been critical in increasing the health of patients. The psychologist is an able professional with research training and experience who is often perceived as a valuable member of hospital committees. Psychologists are well trained to contribute to utilization review, quality improvement, program evaluation, and continuing education committees. Often, the psychologist has background and training in personnel evaluation and selection, organizational management and planning, public relations, and social and group systems. The psychologist is a valuable practitioner dealing with special populations such as substance abusers, children, patients experiencing domestic violence or significant family conflicts, and the terminally ill.

In many communities the rural hospital has come to depend on the expertise and commitment of their rural psychologists. The evolution of the practice of rural hospital psychology has set the stage for an exciting new era of psychologist–physician collaboration and opportunities for rewarding multidisciplinary practice emanating from the rural hospital.

References

American Medical Association. (1991). Statements on delineation of hospital privileges. Chicago: Author.

American Psychological Association. (1985). *A hospital practice primer for psychologists*. Washington, DC: Author.

American Psychological Association. (1991). *Guidelines on hospital privileges: Credentialing and bylaws*. Washington, DC: Author.

American Psychological Association, Office of Demographic, Employment, and Educational Research. (1989). *Employment characteristics of members by type of APA membership: 1989*. Washington, DC: Author.

Baker, F., Jodrey, D., Intagliatia, J., & Straus, H. (1993). Community support services and functioning of the seriously mentally ill. *Community Mental Health Journal, 29*, 321–331.

Bennett, C. C. (1965). Community psychology: Impressions of the Boston Conference on the Education of Psychologists for Community Mental Health. *American Psychologist, 20*, 382–385.

Bennett, C. C., Anderson, L. S., Cooper, S., Hassol, L., Klein, D. C., & Rosenblum, G. (Eds). (1966). *Community psychology: A report of the Boston Conference on the Education for Psychologists in Community Mental Health*. Boston: Boston University Press.

Bersoff, D. N. (1983). Hospital privileges and antitrust laws. *American Psychologist, 45*, 1313–1315.

Bootzin, R. R., Shadish, W. R., & McSweeny, A. J. (1989). Longitudinal outcomes of nursing home care for severely mentally ill patients. *Journal of Social Issues, 45*, 31–48.

Borges, W. J., Summers, L. C., & Karshmer, J. (1995). Psychiatric emergency service. Using available resources. *Journal of Nursing Administration, 25*, 31–37.

Brody, D. S. (1996). What is the role of the primary care physician in managed mental health care? In A. Lazarus (Ed.), *Controversies in managed mental health care*. Washington, DC: American Psychiatric Press.

CAPP v. Rank, 51 Cal.3d 1, 793 P.2d 2 (1990).

Carr, J. E. (1987). Federal impact on psychology in medical schools. *American Psychologist, 42*, 869–872.

Cullen, E. A. (1993). Analysis of existing hospital practice laws for psychologists. Washington, DC: American Psychological Association.

Dafter, R., & Freeland, G. (1988, December). Psychologists' unrealized power in the mental health marketplace. *California Psychologist, 6*, 14.

Dorken, H., Stapp, J., & VandenBos, G. (1986). Licensed psychologists: A decade of major growth. In H. Dorken & associates (Eds.), *Professional psychology in transition: Meeting today's challenges* (pp. 3–19). San Francisco: Jossey-Bass.

Durell, J., Lechtenberg, B., Corse, S., & Frances, R. (1993). Alcohol and drug abuse: Intensive case management of persons with chronic mental illness who abuse substances. *Hospital and Community Psychiatry, 44*, 415–416, 428.

Elefant, A. B. (1985). Psychotherapy and assessment in hospital settings: Ideological and professional conflicts. *Professional Psychology: Research and Practice, 16*, 55–63.

Enright, M. F., & Blue, B. A. (1989). Collaborative treatment of panic disorders by psychologists and family physicians. *Psychotherapy in Private Practice, 7*, 85–90.

Enright, M. F., Resnick, R. J., DeLeon, P. H., Sciara, A. D., & Tanney, F. (1990). The practice of psychology in hospital settings. *American Psychologist, 45*, 1059–1065.

Enright, M. F., Resnick, R. J., Ludwigsen, K. R., & DeLeon, P. H. (1993). Hospital practice: Psychology's call to action. *Professional psychology: Research and Practice, 24*, 135–141.

Fink, P. J. (1986). Dealing with psychiatry's stigma. *Hospital and Community Psychiatry, 37*, 814–818.

Gaylin, S. (1985). The coming of the corporation and the marketing of psychiatry. *Hospital and Community Psychiatry, 36*, 154–159.

Health Care Financing Administration. (1989). 42 C.F.R. Ch IV, Subpart A, P. 310.

Joint Commission on Accreditation of Healthcare Organizations. (1985). *Accreditation manual for hospitals*. Chicago: Author.

Joint Commission on Accreditation of Healthcare Organizations. (1991). *Accreditation manual for hospitals*. Chicago: Author

Joint Commission on Accreditation of Healthcare Organizations. (1992). *Accreditation manual for hospitals: 1992.* Chicago: Author.

Korchin, S. J. (1976). *Modern clinical psychology principles of intervention in the clinic and community.* New York: Basis Books.

Litwin, W. J., Boswell, D. L., & Kraft, W. A. (1991). Medical staff membership and clinical privileges: A survey of hospital-affiliated psychologists. *Professional Psychology: Research and Practice, 22,* 322–327.

Ludwigsen, K. R. (1992). Philosophical and practical issues in pharmacotherapy. *Independent Practitioner, 12,* 180–184.

Ludwigsen, K. R. (1993). Advocacy issues in hospital practice. *Independent Practitioner, 13,* 159–161.

Ludwigsen, K. R., & Albright, D. G. (1994). Training psychologists for hospital practice: A proposal. *Professional Psychology: Research and Practice, 25,* 241–246.

Manderscheid, R. W., & Sonnenschein, M. A. (Eds.). (1991). *Mental health, United States: 1990* (NIMH Publication No. ADM 90-708). Washington, DC: U.S. Government Printing Office.

Matarazzo, J. D., Lubin, B., & Nathan, R. G. (1978). Psychologists' membership on the medical staffs of university teaching hospitals. *American Psychologist, 33,* 23–29.

McCarrick, A. K., Rosenstein, M. J., Milamzo-Sayre, L. J., & Manderscheid, R. W. (1988). National trends in use of psychotherapy in psychiatric inpatient settings. *Hospital and Community Psychiatry, 39,* 835–841.

McLellan, A. T., Arndt, I. O., Metzger, D. S., Woody, G. E., & O'Brien, C. P. (1993). The effects of psychosocial services in substance abuse treatment. *JAMA, 269,* 1953–1959.

Mickel, C. (1982). Innovative projects earning psychologists spots on hospital healthcare teams. *American Psychologist, 37,* 1350–1354.

Morris, J. A. (1995). Alcohol and other drug dependency treatment: A proposal for integration with primary care. *Alcoholism Treatment Quarterly, 13*(3), 45–56.

Mozdzierz, G. J., Snodgrass, R. W., & DeLeon, P. H. (1992). A new role for psychologists: Hospital ethics committees. *Professional Psychology: Research and Practice, 23,* 493–499.

Nielsen, A. C., & Williams, T. A. (1980, September). Depression in ambulatory medical patients. *Archives of General Psychiatry, 37,* 999–1004.

Omnibus Budget Reconciliation Act of 1988, Sec. 4201-4206, 4211-4216, 101 Stat 1330-160 through 1330-220, 42 U.S.C Sec. 1395i-3(a)–(h) [Medicare] and 1396r (a)–(h) [Medicaid] 1992.

Patterns of Psychological Practice Survey. (1984, February). *California State Psychologist, 1,* 3–4.

Pope, K. S. (1990). Ethical and malpractice issues in hospital practice. *American Psychologist, 45,* 1066–1070.

Regier, D. A., Goldberg, I. D., & Taube, C. A. (1978). The de facto U.S. mental health services system: A public perspective. *Archives of General Psychiatry, 35,* 685–693.

Resnick, R. J. (1985). A case against the Blues: The Virginia challenge. *American Psychologist, 39,* 988–995.

Schlesinger, M., & Dorwart, R. (1984). Ownership and mental health services: A reappraisal of the shift toward privately owned facilities. *The New England Journal of Medicine, 311,* 959–965.

Schulberg, H. C., Saul., M., McClelland, M., et al. (1985, December). Assessing depression in primary medical and psychiatric practices. *Archives of General Psychiatry, 42,* 1164–1170.

Schulberg, H. C., & Scott, C. P. (1991). Depression in primary care: Treating depression with interpersonal psychotherapy. In C. S. Austad & W. H. Berman (Eds.), *Psychotherapy in managed health care: The optimal use of time and resources* (pp. 153–170). Washington, DC: American Psychological Association.

Social Security Administration. (1993). Sec. 1861(f), 42 U.S.C. 1395x. *Compilation of the Social Security laws* (Committee Print WMCP:103-5). Washington, DC: U.S. Government Printing Office.

Sweet, J. J., Rozensky, R. H., & Tovian, S. M. (Eds.). (1991). *Handbook of clinical psychology in medical settings* (pp. 59–80). New York: Plenum Press.

Thompson, R. J. (1987). Psychologists in medical schools: Medical staff status and clinical privileges. *American Psychologist, 42,* 866–868.

Thompson, R. J., & Matarazzo, J. D. (1984). Psychology in United States medical schools: 1983. *American Psychologist, 39,* 988–995.

VandenBos, G. R., DeLeon, P. H., & Belar, C. D. (1991). How many psychologists are needed? It's too early to know! *Professional Psychology: Research and Practice, 22,* 441–448.

Zaro, J. S., Batchelor, W. F., Ginsberg, M. R., & Pallak, M. S. (1982). Psychology and the JCAHO: Reflections on a decade of struggle. *American Psychologist, 37,* 1342–1349.

2

Medical or Professional Staff Membership and Participation in Rural Hospitals

Ronald H. Rozensky

The purpose of this chapter is twofold. The first section presents information to help hospital or health care system executives and administrators understand the place of psychologists within the professional or medical staff of the hospital. The second section acquaints the practicing psychologist with the issues surrounding the attainment of hospital medical staff membership and privileges.

To the Hospital Administrator: Psychologists Within Medical Settings

Licensed psychologists practice within a wide range of hospital and health care settings across the country. This reflects the discipline's broad scope of practice. Psychologists are found in private medical–surgical hospitals, private psychiatric facilities, chemical dependency facilities, physical rehabilitation hospitals, public medical hospitals, and public mental health hospitals (Enright, Resnick, DeLeon, Sciara, & Tanney, 1990). The actual clinical privileges of those psychologists are defined by the ethical standards of professional psychology, psychology's educational and training guidelines, and legal regulations controlling the health care environment. Psychologists are reimbursed by third-party payors for all services they provide within their defined scope of practice. Although the distribution of doctoral-level mental health professionals outside of urban environments is routinely low, Murray (1989) found that psychologists are better represented than psychiatrists in rural settings. Furthermore, psychologists "are often the most highly trained mental health and substance abuse professionals in their [rural] communities" (Bray & Rogers, 1995, p. 132).

Hospital Accreditation

Hospital executives and administrators, professional or medical staff members, nursing staff, allied health care providers, and members of the hospital's board of directors alike all know and understand the importance of receiving and maintaining accreditation by the Joint Commission on Accreditation of Healthcare Organizations (JCAHO).

The JCAHO is a private, nonprofit corporation that was developed for the purpose of setting standards for hospitals.

> This particular organization is important because as hospitals are able to meet these standards they are then able to be reimbursed by both third-party and governmental payers for the services they provide. Without these standards being met, most hospitals could not practice because most third-party payers would be reluctant or unable to pay an institution that does not meet JCAH[O] standards. (Committee on Professional Practice of the Board of Professional Affairs, 1985, p. 15)

Thus, the JCAHO sets the national standards to which all quality health care organizations aspire. First and foremost, the JCAHO, since 1983, has permit medical staff membership to include physicians and "other licensed individuals permitted by law and by the hospital to provide patient care services independently in the hospital" (JCAHO, 1992, p. 53). Thus, psychologists, as autonomously licensed health care professionals in all jurisdictions in the United States, are recognized by the JCAHO as independent members of hospital medical staffs. In addition, since 1988, the American Psychological Association (APA) has had a representative on the Behavioral Health Professional and Technical Advisory Committee of the JCAHO. (The author of this chapter served in that capacity from 1993 through 1996.) That committee oversees preparation and review of all mental health care standards for all types of health care facilities and hospitals. Thus, American psychology has an equal voice along with all health care disciplines in both setting national standards of care and in reviewing and monitoring of proposed standards of care in any and all health care organizations.

For any health care executive who might wonder about the legal or accreditation effect of having psychologists on staff, the following standards from the JCAHO's (1992) *Accreditation Manual for Hospitals* clearly permit the hospital practice activities of properly credentialed and privileged licensed psychologists.

M.S.1.1 The medical staff has the following characteristics:

M.S.1.1.1 It includes fully licensed physicians and may include other licensed individuals permitted by law and by the hospital to provide patient care services independently in the hospital.

individual permitted to provide patient care services independently .... any individual who is permitted by law and who is also permitted by the hospital to provide patient care services without direction or supervision, within the scope of his/her license and in accordance with individually granted clinical privileges. Clinical privileges are based on criteria established by the hospital.

M.S.1.1.2 All its members have delineated clinical privileges that allow them to provide patient care services independently within the scope of their clinical privileges.

clinical privileges .... permission to provide medical

or other patient care services in the granting institution, within well-defined limits, based upon the individual's professional license and his/her experience, competence, ability, and judgment. (p. 53)

An even more recent explication of the increasing recognition of the scope of practice for psychologists in hospitals can be found in the 1995 edition of the JCAHO accreditation manual (JCAHO, 1995). For example, Standard HR.1.2 states that the organization should have a process to ensure the competence of all licensed independent practitioners through granting of clinical privileges. Herein, a licensed independent practitioner is "any individual permitted by law and by the organization to provide patient care services without direction or supervision, within the scope of the individual's licensure" (p. 372). Furthermore, the review of competence (HR.1.2.1.4, p. 373) and the granting of clinical privileges (HR.1.2.1.5, p. 373) states that "peer participation is part of the privileging process" (p. 373). Thus, as independent licensed providers, psychologists must be involved, as peers, in the credentialing and privileging of other psychologists. Psychologists are also defined by the JCAHO as "qualified individuals" (JCAHO, 1995, p. 109) and, as such, can "plan and provide care, treatment, or rehabilitation specific to an individual's [patient's] problems and needs" (p. 109). Along with treatment planning and direct care, psychologists can be the "individual permitted by law" (JCAHO, 1995; TX.6.1.4, p. 185) to order or justify such procedures as restraint and seclusion and can serve in clinical leadership roles in the hospital: "clinical leaders include, at least clinical psychologists, psychiatric nurses, psychiatrists, social workers" (JCAHO, 1995; LD.1.8.1, p. 287). The JCAHO states that "clinical leaders participate in determining what qualifications (training, experience, and documented competence) are required for assuming specific clinical service responsibilities" (p. 288). To summarize then, psychologists, as legally recognized independent providers, are able, according to JCAHO standards, to serve as clinical leaders in the hospital, privilege themselves in the peer review process of credentialing, work independently in areas of treatment planning and direct service, and even write orders such as those that justify patient restraint.

When a licensed psychologist requests his or her place on a medical staff, the JCAHO requires first that state law permit or not restrict such membership and then that the hospital establish proper credentialing and privileging mechanisms for the psychologist as it does for any licensed independent provider, physician, or other member of the medical staff.

State and Federal Laws and Hospital Practice

Psychology Licensing. Psychologists are independently licensed health care providers in all jurisdictions of the United States. As such, each state establishes a legal scope of practice for psychologists on the basis of their education and training. Hospital-based practice is clearly included in the education and clinical training of licensed psychologists. Its inclusion within the discipline's scope of practice, on a state-by-state basis, is determined by statute or regulation.

Insurance and Reimbursement: Freedom of Choice. Licensed psychologists are recognized across the country in "freedom of choice" laws that require that health insurers directly recognize and reimburse, for all covered services, psychologists practicing within the scope of their licensure, without the need for referral, supervision, or billing by any other professional. These freedom of choice laws assure that the consumer has the right to select the qualified mental health provider she or he feels can best address her or his health care needs. They also guarantee that psychologists will be reimbursed for their services.

Hospital Licensing and Psychological Practice. Each state has promulgated laws that define or regulate the operation of hospitals within that state. Hospitals clearly must follow these laws and other rules and regulations put forward by departments of health, mental health, or professional regulation. At this time 16 states and the District of Columbia have specific statutes or regulations that require hospitals to permit psychologists to become members of hospital medical staff. Other states stand silent on this issue and, thus, not limiting such membership, permit hospital credentialing to go forward. Both the health care executive and psychologist seeking membership on a hospital's medical staff must be aware of the legal status in his or her state regarding hospital professional staff membership. No matter what the legal environment, the health care administrator should know that by 1991, 13% of all psychologists considered hospitals as their primary work setting (Manderscheid & Sonnenschein, 1991), and approximately 60% of all psychology training internships are in hospital settings (Kurz, Fuchs, Dabek, Kurz, & Helfrich, 1982). Thus, the hospital environment is a natural home for practicing psychologists.

Medicare and Medicaid. Since 1989, Medicare law has permitted psychologists to oversee hospital care of their own Medicare patients. Enactment of 1994 Social Security Act Amendments has clarified questions of Medicare Conditions of Participation now removing any question of psychologists' legal ability to provide continuity of care for their Medicare patients directing their care and following them for treatment both as inpatient attending providers and outpatient care specialists. This clarification of Health Care Financing Administration (HCFA) interpretation now clearly removes any artificial barriers to governmentally or privately funded services for hospital-based psychological practice.

Medicaid provides health care to 32 million low-income adults and children in the United States, with a growing number of elderly and disabled citizens being added yearly to the program (Congressional Research Services, 1993; Sullivan, 1995). Increasingly, federal government waivers are being used by the states to carry out creative research and demonstration projects to use managed care cost-containment mechanisms within Medicaid (Morris, 1994). Currently, psychologists are reimbursed in 50 states for the treatment of Medicaid covered children, adolescents, and families under the congressionally mandated early periodic screening and development programs (HCFA, 1990). As these projects relying on managed-care organizations move forward, psychologists will have the opportunity to be designated as providers in those 25 states where psychologists are yet to be recognized as independent Medicaid providers (Sullivan, 1995). Thus, one should soon see coast-to-coast Medicaid coverage for psychological services. Hospital executives are encouraged to discuss with the psychologist seeking privileges at their hospital the present Medicaid status of psychologists in their state, and to work cooperatively to help add psychological services to appropriate Medicaid rules to ensure that these quality services are available to the widest population.

Psychology's Commitment to Quality Hospital Care: Standards and Ethics

Organized, professional psychology has taken a direct stand on the required competence of hospital practicing psychologists, thus, assuring health care executives and hospital administrators that psychologists on the medical staff of their facilities meet the highest standards of education and training. APA has clear practice guidelines that require proper credentialing and privileging of psychologists within organized health care facilities, as well as ethical standards requiring competence in areas of practice or specialization. APA's policy on hospital privileging of psychologists states that

> It is the policy of the American Psychological Association that privileges should be granted and assigned on the basis of each individual psychologist's documented training and/or experience, demonstrated abilities, and current competence. The privileges granted or assigned to each psychologist should be based on his/her respective qualifications. (Resnick, Enright, & Thompson, 1991, p. 1)

The hospital executive can be assured that psychologists practice only within their areas of competence as a matter of ethics. The following excerpt from the extensive *Ethical Principles of Psychologists and Code of Conduct* of APA illustrates this ethical commitment to both competence and quality care:

> Principle A: Competence. Psychologists strive to main-
> tain high standards of competence in their work. They
> recognize the boundaries of their particular competencies
> and the limitations of their expertise. They provide only
> those techniques for which they are qualified by educa-
> tion, training, or experience. (APA, 1992, p. 3)

Thus, those psychologists seeking to practice within the hospital setting are ethically bound to request only those privileges and practice only those techniques for which they are
adequately trained to provide to the consumer.

Consumer Satisfaction and Medical Staff Cooperation

Murstein and Fontaine (1993) found that patient–consumers'
preference for psychologists is on the rise and that consumers
are "almost as comfortable" with psychologists as they are
with their primary care physicians (p. 884). Similarly, when
looking at physician–psychologist cooperation or physician-
as-consumer of psychological services, on the basis of referral
patterns, one finds that physicians are highly likely to use the
services of psychologists. For example, Vasquez, Nath, and
Murray (1988) found that of those family medicine physicians who made mental health referrals, 71% of the referrals
were made to psychologists. Similarly, Pruitt, Elliott, Mc-
Gowan, Koerner, and Mullins (1988) found that physicians
were more inclined to make referrals to psychologists than
to psychiatrists.

It is clear that psychologists are welcome members of the
hospital health care team and the medical staff. Psychologists
in any hospital setting should be in a position to establish
their own credentialing and privileging standards and the
policies and procedures that govern those services. Even the
American Psychiatric Association has written that in setting
practice guidelines within hospital settings, psychiatry
"could not address the nonpsychiatric practitioner, whether

physician or not, since the psychiatrists cannot define the exact training of another discipline" (Wise et al., 1986, p. 8). Thus, as an independently licensed profession, with its own standards and scope of practice that includes hospital-based health care, psychology and psychologists will make excellent members of any hospital or health care organization's quality health care team.

To the Licensed Clinical Psychologist: Seeking Hospital Privileges

There are many resources available to the practicing psychologist seeking formal hospital medical staff membership and clinical privileges. Publications such as the Committee on Professional Practice of the Board of Professional Affairs' two guide books *A Hospital Practice Primer for Psychologists* (1985) and *Hospital Practice: Advocacy Issues* (1988); Resnick et al. (1991) *Guidelines on Hospital Practice Privileges: Credentialing and Bylaws*; Stromberg et al.'s (1988) *The Psychologist's Legal Handbook*; Rozensky's (1991) "Psychologists, Politics, and Hospitals"; and Rozensky, Sweet, and Tovian's (1997) *Psychological Assessment in Medical Settings* offer specific information to help sort through the often complicated hospital practice issues. The first three texts offer forms for documenting and approving the lists of clinical, consulting, and scientific privileges commonly sought by hospital-based psychologists, thus the forms are not repeated in this guidebook. For psychologists seeking membership on general medical–surgical hospital staffs, discussions such as those on medical cost offset, presented in *Promoting Quality Mental Health Benefits* (APA, 1993), would be of great use in talking both with physicians and hospital administrators.

According to Stromberg et al. (1988), acquisition of medical staff membership does not assure an adequate range of clinical roles for the psychologist in a hospital. "Medical staff membership is only an empty vessel of eligibility" (Stromberg et al., 1988, p. 328) into which the delineation of one's clinical privileges are poured. Such privileges are based on an individual's training, experience, and demonstrated competence (Committee on Professional Practice of the Board of Professional Affairs, 1985). The Committee recommends that "psychologists should attempt to gain explicit approval for the services they provide rather than permitting the institution to allow them to function in an informal fashion" (p. 19). First, however, the psychologists should be aware of the hospital's specific bylaws.

Hospital Bylaws

Hospital bylaws are public documents available through the hospital's board of directors, medical staff officers, or hospital administration. The bylaws define the hospital's mission and set forth the rules for membership access to the professional staff. Thus, the psychologist seeking hospital staff membership should review this document in preparation for discussion with the hospital leadership. Clearly understanding the rules of the game will make the psychologist an informed player. If modification of existing bylaws is necessary to allow the psychologist to be privileged in a hospital, collaboration with colleagues on the medical staff, in hospital administration, and on the hospital board may be required. Such modifications will allow the hospital and psychologist to offer to the public the highest quality psychological services within the broad scope of practice of psychology.

Criteria for Privileging

Permissible Criteria. Hospitals can lawfully grant or decline staff membership and privileges to psychologists "on any basis which is rationally related to his or her competence" (Stromberg et al., 1988, p. 329). The following are criteria that Stromberg et al. stated are permissible as part of the evaluation process for membership and privileging:

1. required information that includes education, internship, fellowships or other training, experience, current competence and licensure, and health status

2. pending or completed professional liability actions or loss of membership or privileges at other institutions

3. academic or educational criteria if clearly related to professional competence (Requirements for psychologists to have a doctoral degree from an accredited educational institution and a documented amount of training and experience are seen as fair criteria in the application process.)

4. requirements to carry a certain amount of malpractice insurance to protect the hospital and members of the professional staff from "having to bear a disproportionate share of any costs stemming from a malpractice claim involving an inadequately insured practitioner" (Stromberg et al., 1988, p. 331)

5. a set geographic limit on staff members' residency to assure that patients can be attended to adequately in an emergency

6. denial of privileges to those whose abilities to work with others or whose personal style can be documented to jeopardize quality of care

7. a "closed staff policy" wherein the entire hospital staff or a given department staff is closed to membership because "the hospital's facilities are not adequate to treat the patients that are likely to be admitted by additional staff members, or that the existing staff is sufficient to meet the hospital's needs" (Stromberg et al., 1988, p. 332). (To avoid antitrust problems in this area, the hospital must be able to document its rationale for such procedures.)

8. observed and documented competency to provide that clinical privileges sought are legitimate measures to assure quality of care.

Nonpermissible Criteria for Privileging. According to Stromberg et al. (1988), there are several criteria that are not permissible for a hospital to use during the application or privileging process, including the following: (a) Membership in professional societies, recommendations of a member of the present professional staff, or affiliation with a certain health maintenance organization (HMO), (b) Age, sex, race, or handicap; and (c) A key question is whether hospitals are free to deny staff membership and privileges to all psychologists as a category. State law varies on this question, with some states allowing such exclusion, others mandating non-discrimination against psychologists, and still others silent on the issue (Stromberg et al., 1988, p. 334).

It is recommended that "in areas where state law does not expressly allow the blanket exclusion of psychologists, a challenge to such a policy may be brought on antitrust or other grounds" (Stromberg et al., 1988, p. 334).

The Privileging Process

According to Stromberg et al. (1988), the application process should provide the psychologist reasonable, written notice of the results of the action. Decisions should be based on stated credentialing and privileging criteria and the information presented by the applicant. Should the applicant question the outcome, there should exist a right to an appeal process.

A committee of peers, other psychologists working in the medical setting, must adjudicate applications for their own discipline and advise the hospital credentialing committee. This should assure the most credible review of a psychologist's credentials. If a peer committee does not exist, it should be requested. The JCAHO (1995) requires (Standard HR.1.2.1.5) that "peer participation is part of the privileging process" (p. 373).

If the psychologist receives an adverse decision, Stromberg et al., (1988) suggested that "the first step should be to examine the basis for the proposed decision and to consider (with counsel) what procedural steps are available to oppose or appeal the decision" (p. 338). The first appeal should be carried out within the hospital's own appeal mechanisms. Only if that fails should legal action proceed.

If there is an organized department, division, or section of psychology in the medical setting in which the psychologist is seeking privileges, seek out the chairperson, director, or chief of that program. Ask for a meeting to discuss the role of the psychology program in that institution. If there is no formal program, seek out either the formal or informal senior psychologist with whom to discuss the role of psychology in that institution. Discussion can focus on one's particular expertise and experience and how that expertise can compliment the existing program. If there is no such formal or informal structure, seek out the existing mental health structure or psychiatry or social work services (with JCAHO standards in hand). Working within the mental health disciplines, at least initially, will help establish the range and level of services that exist within that system.

If that mental health hierarchy does not exist, or is openly hostile to the psychologist's efforts to seek privileges, direct communication with the hospital president, administrative director, or hospital attorney would be appropriate using the material presented earlier in this chapter. The ultimate goals, of course, would be (a) establishing an independent psychology service or department while (b) educating key decision makers about the contributions that psychologists are making in hospital settings and (c) the ultimate formation of ongoing collaborative relationships (Bray & Rogers, 1995).

Once the appropriate initial contact person has been identified, then a meeting to review the hospital's actual requirements for a psychologist to become a member of the professional staff is useful. Discussing the hospital's criteria and one's individual credentials on an informal basis helps acquaint the psychologist with the hospital and the hospital professional staff with the psychologist and service he or she can provide. Should there be any difficulty with one's particular credentials meeting the stated criteria at this point, the credentials can be discussed to help put the application in order prior to the beginning of the formal process.

Practicing With Commitment and Responsibility

The psychologist should be aware of any requirements of members of the professional staff and determine his or her willingness to meet those expectations. For example, professional staff dues, voluntary teaching time, or services in a clinic may be required of all professional staff members. If the medical setting is a teaching facility with formal training programs for psychologists, psychiatrists, or family practitioners, one may be required to meet an academic standard of the parent medical school or university before acceptance on the staff is considered. The psychologist should acquaint himself or herself with those academic requirements, if they exist, to determine a priori both his or her qualifications for an academic appointment and the institution's or training program's actual need for the psychologist's academic services.

Finally, the psychologist should spend time understanding the extent of the actual privileges available to psychologists in the medical setting in question. If physicians' orders or co-signature is necessary for practice, for example, the psychologist must decide if she or he wishes to practice with those restrictions on his or her autonomy. If a psychologist is expecting, for example, to hospitalize his or her patients but this is not a privilege available to psychologists, he or she should discuss to what extent that rule is mutable and to what extent challenging that rule will be accepted by the present psychology department or division. It is certainly easier to change rules from within an organization than to enter anew and challenge the existing establishment without a full appreciation of the institution's history as it pertains to the role and function of clinical psychology.

Specificity of Credentials and Privileges

The psychologist seeking privileges in any hospital or organized medical setting should not respond to the previously listed requirements in a defensive manner or feel burdened any more than any other staff member in the hospital. All members of a medical staff must meet similar criteria and credentialing and privileging requirements put forth by their discipline or department. The neurosurgeon is privileged in the operating room for neurosurgery and is not permitted to use the proctoscope unless specifically qualified and privileged to do so. Thus, the psychologist should step forward with a list of specific privileges sought and the required credentials of education, training, and experience necessary to receive the privilege to carry out each of those specific activities in the hospital. For example, for privileges in neuropsychological assessment, specification of course work, number of supervised cases, and level of training of the supervisors of those cases offer a specific definition of which psychologist is qualified to carry out these assessments. Similarly, for each of the major services provided by psychologists in the institution (e.g., personality assessment, medical or health psychology consultation on medical or surgical units, group psychotherapy, individual psychotherapy, treatment of children vs. adults, biofeedback, or hypnosis) a specific privilege should be defined stating, a priori, each required, documented credential necessary to carry out the services. Importantly, although the right to independently admit and discharge patients is an important privilege, there is a wider range of activities, such as the right to do independent consultations or to attend patients in the emergency room, that may be equally significant in assuring full staff privileges to work with patients.

With the legal right to practice in hospitals comes the ethical responsibility to specify both the academic curriculum and "hands on" training that prepares psychologists for management of inpatients in the psychiatric milieu or to provide treatment of medical patients in any general hospital practice. This requirement to specify credentials is a natural result of admittance into the hospital milieu as independent practitioners; it is part of the rules and can serve as a chance to highlight the scope of practice of psychology, its scientific basis, and its clinical competence to physician colleagues and hospital executives alike.

Thompson (1987) warned that the challenge of delineating and then utilizing clinical privileges "will sorely test the maturity of psychology" (p. 868). Hospital-based psychologists cannot avoid external scrutiny of their practice given the requirements of quality improvement and assurance within the hospital milieu. What better way to communicate to the hospital staff the wide scope of practice for which psychologists are trained.

Conclusion

Psychologists practice in a wide range of organized health care settings. Practice within those settings requires involvement in a system that demands standards of practice and specificity of credentials in a manner quite different from the independence and self-policing of independent office practice. Involvement in hospital practice, however, assures that psychologists' patients will receive adequate continuity of care, that managed-care systems will recognize psychologists' practices as part of larger health care delivery systems, and that psychology's knowledge base and expertise will be available to help ensure quality of care within those systems. Psychologists fit naturally in medical staff membership, and individual health care systems must be approached in a direct, forthright manner to assure psychologists' inclusion as fully recognized, independent providers of health care.

In rural areas, psychologists may be the only qualified behavioral health experts available to hospitalized patients. Responsible advocacy that eradicates barriers to patient choice of doctor, access to psychological services, and improvement of behavioral health services is often a pressing concern of rural psychologists, hospital administrators, and informed medical staff members. Rural psychologists concerned with the quality of care in their local hospital often become meaningful, viable leaders in quality improvement, program development, and medical or professional staff education.

References

American Psychological Association. (1992). Ethical principles of psychologists and code of conduct. *American Psychologist, 12,* 1597–1611.

American Psychological Association. (1993). *Promoting quality mental health benefits.* Washington, DC: Author.

Bray, J. H., & Rogers, J. C. (1995). Linking psychologists and family physicians for collaborative practice. *Professional Psychology: Research and Practice, 26,* 132–138.

Committee on Professional Practice of the Board of Professional Affairs. (1985). *A hospital practice primer for psychologists.* Washington, DC: American Psychological Association.

Committee on Professional Practice of the Board of Professional Affairs. (1988). *Hospital practice: Advocacy issues.* Washington, DC: American Psychological Association.

Congressional Research Services. (1993). *Medicaid source book: Background data and analysis* (Committee Print 103©A). Washington, DC: U.S. Government Printing Office.

Enright, M. F., Resnick, R., DeLeon, P. H., Sciara, A. D., & Tanney, F. (1990). The practice of psychology in hospital settings. *American Psychologist, 45,* 1059–1065.

Health Care Financing Administration. (1990, April). *Early and periodic screening, diagnosis and treatment (EPSDT), state medicaid manual* (HCFA ©Pub. 45-5, Transmittal No. 3, PB90-952601). Washington, DC: HCFA.

Joint Commission on Accreditation of Healthcare Organizations. (1992). *Accreditation manual for hospitals (1993).* Oakbrook Terrace, IL: Author.

Joint Commission on Accreditation of Healthcare Organizations. (1995). *Accreditation manual for mental health, chemical dependency, and mental retardation/developmental disabilities services.* Oakbrook Terrace, IL: Author.

Kurz, R. B., Fuchs, M., Dabek, R. F., Kurz, S. M. S., & Helfrich, W. T. (1982). Characteristics of predoctoral internships in professional psychology. *American Psychologist, 37,* 1213–1220.

Manderscheid, R. W., & Sonnenschein, M. A. (Eds.). (1991). *Mental health, United States: 1990* (NIMH Publication No. ADM 90©708). Washington, DC: U.S. Government Printing Office.

Morris, J. A. (1994). The history of managed care and its impact on psychodynamic treatment. *Journal of Psychoanalysis and Psychotherapy, 11,* 129–137.

Murray, J. D. (1989). *The distribution of licensed psychologists and psychiatrists in Pennsylvania: A brief report.* Unpublished manuscript, Mansfield University, Rural Services Institute, Mansfield, PA.

Murstein, B. I., & Fontaine, P. A. (1993). The public's knowledge about psychologists and other mental health professionals. *American Psychologist, 48,* 839–845.

Pruitt, S., Elliott, C., McGowan, R., Koerner, K., & Mullins, L. (1988, August). *Physician referral patterns as impediments to collaboration in behavioral medicine.* Paper presented at the 96th Annual Convention of the American Psychological Association, Atlanta, GA.

Resnick, R. J., Enright, M. F., & Thompson, R. J. (1991). *Guidelines on hos-*

pital practice privileges: Credentialing and bylaws. Washington, DC: American Psychological Association.

Rozensky, R. H. (1991). Psychologists, politics, and hospitals. In J. J. Sweet, R. H. Rozensky, & S. M. Tovian, (Eds.), Handbook of clinical psychology in medical settings (pp. 59–80). New York: Plenum.

Rozensky, R. H., Sweet, J. J., & Tovian, S. M. (1997). *Psychological assessment in medical settings.* New York: Plenum.

Stromberg, C. D., Haggarty, D. J., Leibenluft, R. F., McMillian, M. H., Mishkin, B., Rubin, B. L., & Trilling, H. R. (1988). *The psychologist's legal handbook.* Washington, DC: Council for the National Register of Health Service Providers in Psychology.

Sullivan, M. J. (1995). Medicaid's quiet revolution: Merging the public and private sectors of care. *Professional Psychology: Research and Practice, 26,* 229–234.

Thompson, R. J. (1987). Psychologists in medical schools: Medical staff status and clinical privileges. *American Psychologist, 42,* 866–868.

Vasquez, A., Nath, C., & Murray, S. (1988). Counseling by family physicians: Report of a survey and curriculum modifications in West Virginia. *Family Systems Medicine, 6,* 463–466.

Wise, T. N., Miller, R. D., Rada, R., Barter, J. T., Wallach, H., & Hammersley, D. W. (1986). *Credentials and privileges for psychiatrists in hospital-based practice.* Washington, DC: American Psychiatric Association.

Psychology's Contribution to the Hospital During the Industrialization of Health Care

Jerry A. Morris

A ny discussion of hospital practice must address the immense changes that have been occurring in hospitals since the 1970s. Managed care and the trend toward the industrialization of health care have drastically altered the practices of hospitals and the relationships of the medical staff to them. This chapter reviews the history of how psychology has fared within, and responded to, the managed-care revolution, and it provides a series of recommendations that both hospital administrators and psychologists can adopt for thriving in the new managed-care environment.

Managed-Care Modifications of Infrastructure

Managed-care systems began to focus on the management of costs in the 1970s (Bengen, 1993). Cost savings were sought through prepaid health plans, with guaranteed limits on total costs; a reduced number of approved practitioners to educate, monitor, and supervise; and group practice service delivery designed to minimize overhead and maximize the uniformity of service delivery (Bittker, 1992). These systems, foreign to the traditions of private practice, were touted as the "new industrialization" by some who embraced them and became involved in their dissemination (Bevan, 1982; Cummings, 1986; Cummings & Fernandez, 1985).

It is clear that this new industrialization was not aimed at behavioral health services but rather was aimed at curbing what some deemed excessive diagnostic and medical interventions, and hospital and drug costs (Sperry, 1993), under the concept of "medical or clinical necessity." Initially, mental health services were considered too costly to incorporate in the mainstream of controlled health care programs and were generally made optional (Public Health Service Act, 1992). Certainly, hospital mental health services were considered costly, with 70% of the mental health dollar being spent on inpatient services (Stanton, 1989) and the majority of this covering inpatient adolescent and substance abuse services.

By the late 1970s, health maintenance organizations (HMOs) could not become federally qualified unless they included crisis-intervention mental health services, alcohol and drug detoxification, and referral services for alcohol and drug abuse (Health Maintenance Organization Act of 1973, 1981; Health Maintenance Organization Amendment of 1976). This event made hospitals, and consequently behavioral health units and services in hospitals, a primary target for utilization review, barriers to access, and demands for short lengths of stay.

During the initial nonprofit stage of development, managed-care organizations adopted the philosophy of attempting to organize, finance, deliver, and evaluate health service in a manner that deliberately sought to control costs while providing high-quality health care. They publicly touted an approach that attempted to control costs while delivering high-quality health care and thus conceptually sought to balance availability, access, utilization, and cost on the basis of established clinical need and proven efficacy of selected and approved interventions. The organized systems of care all adopted goals of (a) containing costs, (b) coordinating access to appropriate services, and (c) achieving high-quality outcomes for service recipients.

The ability of managed care to reach these lofty goals rests in the dynamic interplay between stockholder pressures for profits, asset accumulation, and dividends, and the provision of services that maintain consumer health and well-being.

As the control of organized systems of care shifted to private for-profit organizations, many watchful eyes were scanning data to ascertain the extent that these humanistic goals could be maintained (Morris, 1994). Early outcome data on the effectiveness of managed-care approaches have resulted in mixed reviews (Des Harnais, 1985; Fruend et al., cited in Congressional Research Service, 1993). Many argue that the relevant and significant variables germane to quality care are not being measured when managed-care companies are evaluated, and psychologists have not developed adequate methodologies and supporting studies to convincingly demonstrate required evaluative schema (DeLeon, VandenBos, & Bulatao, 1983). It has been estimated that the average group practice contracting with managed care will spend 30% to 40% of gross revenue on the time and office systems necessary to meet the reporting requirements of managed-care companies (Stechler, 1996). The hospital psychologist will require an answering service; partners to cover rotations, absences, and vacations; effective secretarial coordination of appointments and commitments in widely fluctuating patient loads; and comprehensive documentation and billing facilities capable of accommodating very short timelines.

Managed care's staunch opposition to the use of hospitalization in all but crisis situations, and then only for brief stabilization, marks a major shift in health care philosophy (Williams, 1996). Some have maintained that such involvement with insurers actively participating in treatment decisions represents a serious threat to the outcome in psychotherapy and establishes a very complex "adaptational context" or "unnecessary adaptation" (Langs, 1979). Others maintain that managed-care-based treatment planning and coverage results in benefits that are neither predictable nor reliable (Meehan, 1996). Old hospital standards seeking maximal safety and state of the art or optimal treatment based on doctor/patient collaboration and trust are being replaced by resource conservation thinking and contract-oriented treatment planning. Whether this approach is based on efficiency and a more appropriate application of "medical and clinical necessity" or is the transition to "minimally adequate" service and safety remains to be proven.

Some argue that corporate entities motivated by customer satisfaction, competition, and profit-driven efficiency can replace the complacency, low productivity, and waste of the public and nonprofit systems (Austad & Berman, 1991). It has been pointed out that the lack of responsiveness of overburdened public systems with waiting lists, guaranteed tax base that extends year after year regardless of performance and consumer satisfaction, and state and federal umbrella regulation that blocks competition and free-market forces cripples the system. The great comparative trial juxtaposing the public, quasi-public, and free-market systems have been set in place, and answers will be emerging over the next several years (Morris, 1996).

While the federal government financially subsidized the HMO industry between 1973 and 1983, when subsidies were discontinued, for-profit HMOs and independent practice associations (IPAs) entered the market place. Within a short time 20% of psychiatric hospitals owned managed-care organizations (Dorwart & Epstein, 1992), and by the late 1980s 53% of HMOs surveyed in a large study were for-profit organizations (Levin & Glasser, 1992). By 1994, for-profit managed-care organizations had taken over control of the health delivery system, with consolidations and mergers of these giant systems permeating the industry (Barron & Sands, 1996).

It had become clear that profit by restricting services as far as reasonably possible had evolved as one of the primary motives of the managed-care system. The modern hospital faced the new industrialization with the greatest armament of diagnostic and life-saving equipment, the most highly skilled providers, and the most sophisticated and demanding patients of all time. However, payors and the government were gearing up to create an atmosphere of distrust among patient, doctor, and facility, and to resist the contractual right of patients to access the optimal and best services with the fecundity to make their own choice (Morris, 1996). It is in this new environment that the hospital must operate and the psychologist must find the leverage to bring access of high-quality inpatient psychological services to their patients.

Managed Care and Hospital Practice

The escalating prevalence of mental illness, which indicates that 57% of all citizens will suffer from a mental disorder in their lifetime, with 20% requiring psychological intervention (Regier et al., 1984); escalating per capita expenditures for health services ("Health Care," 1993); and growing concern and frustration with failed solutions has resulted in the development of alternative systems known as "managed health care" systems (Ellwood, 1988; Faltermeyer, 1988). The first psychology driven managed care company (American Biodyne, now owned by MedCo, a wholly owned subsidiary of Merck) not only flourished during the mid-1970s and early 1980s but became a leader in the industry (Cummings, 1985, 1986).

The transition to organized systems of care on the basis of a restricted understanding of "medical necessity" and a strong preference for outpatient services has resulted in major changes in the hospital industry (Williams, 1996). Although the hospital has served as a "holding environment," providing the safety, opportunity for benign working through, and the establishment of stabilizing relationships (object constancy), even the avid hospital practitioner must acknowledge that it has been one of the most expensive treatments. In fact, hospital and drug costs have been estimated to be approximately 55% of national health care expenditures, whereas outpatient costs for mental health services have remained reasonably stable (Levin & Glasser, 1992). Some data indicate that outpatient care has often proven to be just as effective as inpatient treatment (Morris, 1995). This situation has resulted in a shift of patients away from hospitals, shortened lengths of stay, and significant managed-care resistance to hospitalization as a treatment method

(Eichmann, Griffin, Lyons, Larson, & Finkel, 1992; Morris, 1996).

Although cost-containment measures are dramatically changing the health care delivery system (Bennett, 1986; Berman et al., 1988; Fielding, 1984; Kisch & Austad, 1988; Barron & Sands, 1996), the most affected component of the system is the hospital. Although the traditional hospitalization for individuals with mental illness went up to 90 days in 1985 (Williams, 1996), the current length of stay approved by managed-care companies ranges from 3 to 7 days with a crisis management focus (Cummings, 1991). In addition, changes in reimbursement on the basis of diagnostic related groups (DRGs) rather than the traditional "audited cost plus" system for Medicaid and Medicare (Cummings, 1996), and the resultant cost shifting driving indemnity plan rates up (Morris, 1995), resulted in powerful selection against hospitalization both at the consumer and third-party contractor levels. The results are barriers to inpatient care and consideration of dramatically shortened lengths of stay when hospitalization during crisis is required.

Realistically, short-term approaches to target symptom management and amelioration with intermittent follow-up have demonstrated considerable viability (Cummings, 1991). However, many argue that significant differences may actually exist between the crisis amelioration approach of brief hospitalization and therapy and the enhanced developmental level that is achieved through more intensive growth experiences (Barron & Sands, 1996). Regardless of the theoretical and scientific position of the psychologist practicing in the hospital, or the hospital administration's wishes, the hospital psychologist of the future will, of necessity, have to be capable of providing short-term and crisis-oriented services to be followed up by intensive outpatient care.

The attending psychologist and physician practicing in hospitals will face powerful pressure to quickly diagnose and analyze patients, set modest and achievable goals, mobilize family and community resources prior to discharge, and ensure that adequate outpatient treatment and monitoring is not only available but implemented. Administrators and clinical directors of hospital programs will be under significantly increased liability and community pressure to ensure that patients and pedestrians are safe, that aftercare alternatives are effective, and that a qualified provider is willing to accept responsibility for patients as they are transitioned to outpatient care. Damaged patients already frustrated with feelings of abandonment by the hospital, stressed by the rush through the inpatient and recovery process, and potentially angry at a third-party carrier for exhorting doctors to limit care will become a lightening rod for malpractice juggernauts and aggressive attorneys.

The hospital environment of rapid change, intensified responsibility, and shifting balances of power will create significant opportunities for individuals with psychology training. The psychologist usually has an active outpatient practice, considerable experience in patient monitoring, crisis intervention, and ready accessibility through on-call services and rapid availability of appointments. He or she is generally trained in both short-term behavioral techniques conducive to inpatient crisis management and intensive psychotherapy suited for the acutely ill patient. Many psychologists have considerable family therapy training that can be brought to bear on the hospitalized patient's kin and influence networks with considerable planning and alliance building necessary for short hospital stays.

The psychologist often has considerable experience in the management of psychological problems emerging out of physical illness and crisis (which have been previously treated in the hospital holding environment by maintaining the medicosurgical patient on an inpatient and observed basis until psychological symptoms subside). The outpatient psychologist following discharged patients after brief stays can document the patient's need to return to the hospital when medical noncompliance or clinical deterioration occur and assist the patient and the hospital in negotiations with managed-care entities. In capitated plans, this coordinated case management provided by the psychologist can prevent lengthy hospitalizations resulting in significant cost savings and allows the flexibility to attempt several short hospital stays.

Perhaps the most compelling argument for the inclusion of psychologists on hospital staffs in the managed care era is the necessity of continuity of care. In most rural and many urban areas, the psychologist has prior experience with the patient who needs to be hospitalized. He or she is often familiar with the case or has worked closely with the patient's physician or other provider or may be the ongoing outpatient doctor treating the patient and family. The psychologist may be aware of important diagnostic and treatment planning issues that can dramatically shorten the assessment and inpatient treatment period. For instance, a patient may have an addiction in addition to mental illness such that self-administered or self-monitored medications have not been advisable. A patient may be at risk for suicide, which only emerges during rages when the patient has had to accept "no" for an answer. A patient may have a significant problem with medication noncompliance. In another patient, personality attributes may be present with intense paranoia. The patient may thus have a proclivity to trust and cooperate only with those who have been repeatedly tested and with whom a long-term, though intermittent, relationship exists. Such psychologists are the grounding that will be required to make short-term crisis hospitalizations work.

Managed care and shortened lengths of stay will put increasing pressures on hospital owners, boards, and administrations to increase the volume of hospital placements. A hospital bed that required 1 referred patient every 30 to 90 days to fill will now require 4 to 10 patients each 30 days. Hospitals will be increasingly interested in practitioners who may have need of inpatient services for their patients and who will loyally rehospitalize patients when managed-care companies too early force them into outpatient care.

Managed-care approaches will increasingly rely on medication-based interventions. Mental patients and certain medical patients have notoriously poor medication compliance if not followed by a psychotherapist (Janis, 1984; Krantz & Glass, 1984; Leventhal, Zimmerman, & Gutman, 1984). Evidence is mounting that medication with psychotherapy and psychotherapy alone are superior approaches to medication alone when treating certain types of patients (Antonuccio, Danton, & DeNelsky, 1995). Hospitals entering into capitated and self-insured agreements will take a good look at psychologists inpatient and outpatient follow-up with patients who have shown poor medication and medical compliance, and who have symptoms of chronic and persistent mental illness.

Hospitals will be scanning the practitioner environment for those psychotherapists willing to take on a long-term patient in a short-term funding environment. The hospital will need the psychologist and psychiatrist to commit to take patients on rotation who will need extensive psychotherapy after being discharged. These patients will need a complex holding environment (Winnicott, 1960) in which to improve. This environment can no longer be provided by the hospital with the imposed shortened lengths of stay currently available. The doctor accepting a patient on his or her service in the hospital will, of necessity, need special skills. These patient management skills will include the setting and maintaining of the frame of therapy by controlling and directing a team of professionals and facets of the institution in mobilizing leverage and family and community resources without destroying the therapeutic vessel and patient confidence and trust, and in protecting the patient and community by ensuring patient monitoring and constraint (Rinsley, 1980). Psychologists with strong dynamic and psychoanalytic training, coupled with adaptability and skill at managing complex boundaries and team, family, and institutional relationships, will be in great demand in hospital systems.

More than ever, hospitals will need the services of psychologists with advanced diagnostic skills. Hospitals will be forced into decisions about discharge, placement and referral, the effect of guardianship and involuntary commitment, and selection of treatment approaches earlier and earlier in the treatment of the patient. These decisions are fraught with the potential of negative consequences for the patient, patient's family, practitioner, employers, and the institution. General medical specialists have shown poor capacity to diagnose the underlying mental illness that may influence these decisions (Morris, 1994). The psychologist who is firmly grounded in the developmental and dynamic psychology, with excellent skills in determining the nature of a developmental arrest, the potential types of acting out, and the necessary holding and treatment environments, and engaging the patient in a working relationship that is based on trust and a willingness to tolerate ensuing anxieties and transferences will be invaluable to the patient and hospital.

Hospitals in the managed-care era of the new industrialized health care will not want to treat and discharge these very complex individuals without the full involvement of a talented psychologist or psychiatrist from the point of admission through protracted aftercare. Many psychologists and psychiatrists may be unwilling to assume such commitment and responsibility in the face of a maximum limit of 20 psychotherapy sessions per year, lifetime service limits, and inpatient time and documentation demands. Those who do will be notably appreciated by the hospital and will likely need a close affiliation with an emergency on-call group, group homes, and residential care centers for nonhospital backup.

Recommended Psychologist and Hospital Collaboration

It is highly likely that wise administrators and chiefs of medical staffs will encourage the recruitment of psychologists during the managed-care era. In doing so, they will limit their liability (Williams, 1996), increase the quality and versatility of care, and add the outpatient psychologist as a referral source. Psychologists will need to maintain a skill and practice base that is attractive to the hospital but must understand the responsibilities to the patient, themselves, and society that they are shouldering with the limited tools available within the managed-care environment.

In partnering, both entities will need to be mindful that

successful operations have several basic things in common: (a) a quality product or service, (b) a product that fills a real and perceived need, (c) personnel delivering the product or service who are adequate to the task and are superior to the competition.

It will therefore behoove the hospital to maintain the highest qualified, well-motivated, and professionally committed psychology staff available. It will be incumbent on the hospital psychologist to maintain an active outpatient practice in close proximity to the hospital and to focus basic and continuing education on those skills that will facilitate rapid assessment and diagnosis, crisis intervention and patient management, treatment of the serious and persistently mentally ill, rehabilitation of the psychological facets of physical illness, and intensive outpatient care and case management.

To attract such psychologists, hospitals will need to make by-laws and policies and procedures attractive to the practice of psychology in the inpatient setting. In many states this means participation in medical staff meetings, committees, and governance of the institution.

Psychologists appreciate clear and uniform structure. They enjoy procedural protocols indicating when mental consultation is required on medicosurgical units, emergency rooms, and pre- and postoperatively. They appreciate the delivery of patient-sensitive educational components of care that manage patient fears and anxiety and map out a road to recovery mobilizing patient problem solving, compliance, and participation in one's own care (Dansereau, Joe, & Simpson, 1993; Gelatt, 1989; Husband & Platt, 1993). The psychologist appreciates access to support services such as the doctor's lounge, dining room, parking slots, and medical records and dictation systems. Inclusion in marketing vehicles advertising the medical and professional staff is valued by psychologists. The psychologist enjoys participation in continuing education and is often required to amass a number of hours of such experiences to maintain a license. Most of all, the psychologist enjoys working with institutions and other providers who are ethically committed to the well-being of the patient; who are sensitive to the thoughts, concerns, and values of the patient; and who understand that health is a holistic phenomenon requiring balance of mind, body, and social system with no one of these variables being more important than the other in the maintenance of long-term health (Cohen, 1993). Psychologists enjoy contributing to systems that avoid the strict biomedicalization of illness and eschew tradition and viewpoints that dismiss or ignore scientific data that alludes to proven effective or even necessary psychological interventions (R. Friedman, Sobel, Myers, Caudill, & Benson, 1995).

Conclusion

The managed-care era has changed the nature of hospital practice, resulting in shortened lengths of stay, increased responsibility and stress related to the immediate aftercare period, and pressure to increase medical and psychological compliance. Significant savings may be available if the system is successful in curbing inpatient costs, which make up a large portion of annual health care expenditures. But a major revolution in the way outpatient psychologists and psychiatrists and general physicians practice will need to occur if this process is to be safe and conducive to patient health and recovery.

The system will increasingly rely on practitioners who can formulate rapid assessments and realistic crisis-management treatment plans, establish a therapeutic relationship that can quickly translate to outpatient care, and mobilize and manage family and community resources. It has been said that to prosper in the new organized systems of care the psychologist will need to become a primary rather than a preferred provider (Shueman, Troy, & Mayhugh, 1994) and make the attitudinal adjustments necessary to succeed (S. Friedman & Fanger, 1991). It may be said that hospital administrators and chiefs of medical staffs will need the same willingness to move psychologist providers into the mainstream of hospital operations and make the attitudinal changes necessary to foster the integration of medical and psychological practitioners.

The hospital psychologist is uniquely trained and positioned to fill the emerging need for rapid mental health and behavioral interventions, followed by competent outpatient care. The collaboration of psychologists and administrators will emerge as one of the guideposts for the evaluation of the effectiveness of management by boards and contracted managed-care corporations. The new customer, the employers, overwhelmingly believe that psychological interventions can significantly impact medical and surgical costs (Oss, 1993). The ability of the psychologist to manage patient care within these emerging parameters will determine the rapidity of the emergence of the era of increased accessibility of hospital services.

References

Antonuccio, D. O., Danton, W. G., & DeNelsky, G. Y. (1995). Psychotherapy versus medication for depression: Challenging the conventional wisdom with data. *Professional Psychology: Research and Practice, 26,* 574–585.

Austad, C. S., & Berman, W. H. (Eds.). (1991). *Psychotherapy in managed health care: The optimal use of time and resources.* Washington, DC: American Psychological Association.

Barron, J. W., & Sands, H. (Eds.). (1996). *Impact of managed care on psychodynamic treatment.* Madison, CT: International Universities Press.

Bengen, B. (1993). *Profiting from managed care in the third generation: Strategies for providers of behavioral health and substance abuse services.* Providence, RI: Manisses Communications Group.

Bennett, M. (1986). Maximizing the yield of psychotherapy: Part II. *HMO Mental Health Newsletter, 1,* 1–4.

Berman, W. H., Kisch, J., DeLeon, P. H., Cummings, N. C., Binder, J. L., & Hefele, T. J. (1988). The future of psychotherapy in the age of diminishing resources. *Psychotherapy in Private Practice, 5,* 105–118.

Bevan, W. (1982). Human welfare and national policy: A conversation with Stuart Eizenstat. *American Psychologist, 37,* 1128–1135.

Bittker, T. (1992). The emergence of prepaid psychiatry. In J. L. Feldman & R. J. Fitzpatrick (Eds.), *Managed mental health care, administrative and clinical issues* (pp. 3–10). Washington, DC: American Psychiatric Press.

Public Health Service Act. (1992). Subpart B—Qualified Health Maintenance Organization requirements (42 CRF 417.101). Washington, DC: Office of the Federal Register, National Archives and Records Administration.

Cohen, C. I. (1993). The biomedicalization of psychiatry: A critical overview. *Community Mental Health Journal, 29,* 509–521.

Congressional Research Service. (1993). Medicaid source book: Background data and analysis. (Committee Print 103-A). Washington, DC: U.S. Government Printing Office.

Cummings, N. A. (1985, August). The new mental healthcare delivery system and psychology's new role. Invited Awards Address presented at the 93rd Annual Convention of the American Psychological Association, Los Angeles.

Cummings, N. A. (1986). The dismantling of our health system: Strategies for the survival of psychological practice. *American Psychologist, 41,* 426–431.

Cummings, N. A. (1991). Brief intermittent therapy throughout the life cycle. In C. S. Austad & W. H. Berman (Eds.), *Psychotherapy in managed health care: The optimal use of time and resources.* Washington, DC: American Psychological Association.

Cummings, N. A. (1996). Behavioral health after managed care: The next golden opportunity for mental health practitioners. In N. A. Cummings, M. S. Pallak, & J. L. Cummings (Eds.), *Surviving the demise of solo practice: Mental health practitioners prospering in the era of managed care* (pp. 27–40). Madison, CT: Psycho-social Press.

Cummings, N. A., & Fernandez, L. (1985, March). Exciting new opportunities for psychologists in the market place. *Independent Practitioner, 5,* 38–42.

Dansereau, D. F., Joe, G. W., & Simpson, D. D. (1993). Node-link mapping: A visual representation strategy for enhancing drug abuse counseling. *Journal of Counseling Psychology, 40,* 385–395.

DeLeon, P. H., VandenBos, G. R., & Bulatao, E. Q. (1983). Psychotherapy: Is it safe, effective, and appropriate? *American Psychologist, 38,* 907–911.

Des Harnais, S. I. (1985). Enrollment in and disenrollment from health maintenance organizations by medicaid recipients. *Health Care Financing Review, 6*(3), 39–50.

Dorwart, R. A., & Epstein, S. S. (1992). Economics and managed mental health care: The HMO as a crucible for cost-effective care. In J. L. Feldman & R. J. Fitzpatrick (Eds.), *Managed mental health care, administrative and clinical issues* (pp. 11–27). Washington, DC: American Psychiatric Press.

Eichmann, M. A., Griffin, B. P., Lyons, J. S., Larson, D. B., & Finkel, S. (1992). An estimation of the impact of OBRA-877 on nursing home care in the United States. *Hospital and Community Psychiatry, 43,* 781.

Ellwood, P. (1988). The Shattuck lecture—Outcomes management: A technology of patient experience. *New England Journal of Medicine, 318,* 1549–1556.

Faltermeyer, E. (1988, October 10). Medical care's next revolution. *Fortune,* 126–130.

Fielding, S. L. (1984). Organizational impact on medicine: The HMO concept. *Social Science and Medicine, 18,* 615–620.

Friedman, R., Sobel, D., Meyers, P., Caudill, M., & Benson, H. (1995). Behavioral medicine, clinical health psychology and cost offset. *Health Psychology, 14,* 509–518.

Friedman, S., & Fanger, M. T. (1991). *Expanding therapeutic possibilities: Getting results in brief psychotherapy.* Lexington, MA: Lexington Books.

Gelatt, H. B. (1989). Positive uncertainty: A new decision-making framework for counseling. *Journal of Counseling Psychology, 36,* 252–256.

Health Care Is Taking a Bigger Bite From Family Budgets; Businesses Are Paying More, Too. (1993, March–April). *Health Beat: Rural Health News Update & Review,* p. 1.

Health Maintenance Organization Act of 1973. Public Law 93-222, 87 STAT. 914, 1973.

Health Maintenance Organization Act of 1981. Public Law 97-35, 95 STAT. 572, 1981.

Health Maintenance Organization Amendment of 1976. Public Law 94-960, 90 STAT. 1945, 1976.

Husband, S. D., & Platt, J. J. (1993). The cognitive skills component in substance abuse treatment in correctional settings: A brief review. *Journal of Drug Issues, 23,* 31–42.

Janis, I. (1984). The patient as decision maker. In D. W. Gentry (Ed.), *Handbook of behavioral medicine* (pp. 326–368). New York: Guilford Press.

Kisch, J., & Austad, C. S. (1988). The health maintenance organization: I. Historical perspective and current status. *Psychotherapy, 25,* 441–448.

Krantz, D. S., & Glass, D. C. (1984). Personality, behavior patterns, and physical illness: Conceptual and methodological issues. In D. W. Gentry (Ed.), *Handbook of behavioral medicine* (pp. 38–86). New York: Guilford Press.

Langs, R. (1979). *The therapeutic environment.* New York: Jason Aronson.

Leventhal, H., Zimmerman, R., & Gutman, M. (1984). Compliance: A Self-regulation perspective. In D. W. Gentry (Ed.), *Handbook of behavioral medicine* (pp. 369–436). New York: Guilford Press.

Levin, B. L., & Glasser, J. H. (1992). Comparing mental health benefits, utilization patterns, and costs. In J. L. Feldman & R. J. Fitzpatrick (Eds.), Managed mental health care, administrative and clinical issues (pp. 29–52). Washington, DC: American Psychiatric Press.

Meehan, B. (1996). From "comfort" to chaos: Mental health insurance coverage in the 1990s. In J. W. Barron & H. Sands (Eds.), *Impact of managed care on psychodynamic treatment* (pp. 73–103). Madison, CT: International Universities Press.

Morris, J. A. (1994). The history of managed care and its impact on psychodynamic treatment. *Journal of Psychoanalysis and Psychotherapy, 11,* 129–137.

Morris, J. A. (1995). Quality standards in corporate dominated health care. *The Independent Practitioner, 15,* 116–119.

Morris, J. A. (1996). The history of managed care and its impact on psychodynamic treatment. In J. W. Barron & H. Sands (Eds.), *Impact of managed care on psychodynamic treatment* (pp. 203–218). Madison, CT: International Universities Press.

Oss, M. (1993, June). The future of occupational medicine. Address presented at the National Workers' Compensation and Occupational Medicine Seminar, Hyannis, MA.

Regier, D. A., Myers, J. K., Kramer, M., Robins, L. N., Blazer, D. G., Hough, R. L., Eaton, W. W., & Locke, B. Z. (1984). The NIMH Epidemiologic Catchment Area program: historical context, major objectives, and study population characteristics. *Archives of General Psychiatry, 41,* 934–941.

Rinsley, D. B. (1980). *Treatment of the severely disturbed adolescent.* New York: Jason Aronson.

Shueman, S. A., Troy, W. G., & Mayhugh, S. L. (1994). Managed behavioral healthcare. *Register Report, 20,* 5–9.

Sperry, P. (1993, May 25). High tech medicine's high cost. *Investor's Business Daily,* pp. 1–2.

Stanton, D. (1989). Mental healthcare economics and the future of psychiatric practice. *Psychiatric Annals, 19,* 421–427.

Stechler, G. (1996). The blind oppressing the recalcitrant: Psychoanalysis, managed care, and family systems. In J. W. Barron & H. Sands (Eds.), *Impact of managed care on psychodynamic treatment* (pp. 181–200). Madison, CT: International Universities Press.

Williams, J. (1996). A holding environment for children in the era of managed care. In J. W. Barron & H. Sands (Eds.), *Impact of managed care on psychodynamic treatment* (pp. 165–179). Madison, CT: International Universities Press.

Winnicott, D. W. (1960). The theory of the parent–infant relationship. *International Journal of Psycho-Analysis, 41,* 585–595.

II

Collaboration and Linkages

Collaboration With Primary Care Physicians

James H. Bray, Michael F. Enright, and John Rogers

With the changing health care market, there is an increased need for psychologists to collaborate with primary care physicians and other medical providers. Particularly in rural areas, primary care physicians are usually the first medical professionals to encounter patients' behavioral health problems (Rakel, 1995).

Unfortunately, psychologists practice in offices that are often isolated from primary care health care providers, and therefore behavioral health problems often go undiagnosed or untreated (Bray & Rogers, 1995; Higgins, 1994; Kroenke & Mangelsdorff, 1989). Many psychologists have little or no training in working with primary care physicians and are not educated about this aspect of the health care system (Bray, 1996; Enright, Resnick, DeLeon, Sciara, & Tanney, 1990).

The Linkages Project—a demonstration project that trained

The Linkages Project was supported by the Center for Substance Abuse Treatment, Substance Abuse and Mental Health Services Administration Contract 92MF05154001D, to the American Psychological Association. Thanks are extended to Gil Hill and Marquette Turner for their help with the project and to the professionals for taking time from their busy practices to participate in the project.

psychologists and family physicians for collaborative practice—provides a training model for psychologists and family physicians to facilitate collaborative practice (Bray & Rogers, 1995). This model focused on treatment of alcohol and other drug abuse problems in rural areas and frontier communities. This chapter reviews the training program and general principles that were learned from this demonstration project (Bray & Rogers, 1997). It also presents basic principles for successful collaborative practice by psychologists and primary care physicians in rural areas (Enright & Blue, 1989). The following issues should be considered when setting up collaborations between psychologists and primary care physicians in rural communities (Bray & Rogers, 1997).

A goal of this program is to develop "generalist" psychologists who are able to collaborate effectively with medical practitioners in rural areas. Training in family systems or contextual theory is particularly useful for this collaboration because it facilitates the mental health provider's ability to take a "broader" viewpoint and negotiate roles and relationships with both physicians and patients (Glenn, 1985; McDaniel, Hepworth, & Doherty, 1992). Psychologists who have been trained in a wide variety of models other than family systems have also benefited from meaningful collaboration.

Theory and Practice of Medicine

Unlike the behavioral health disciplines, medicine uses a unified theory (i.e., the biomedical model on which to base practice). Medical personnel (physicians, nurses, and other support personnel) use a common language for describing and understanding functioning and problems. Familiarity with this language is essential for success in this venue. In addition, it is important to keep in mind that the model of illness is biomedical, which means that medical practitioners look to physical pathology to explain signs, symptoms, and complaints.

Training and "Cultural" Differences Between Psychologists and Physicians

Physicians are indoctrinated throughout their training in a culture quite different from that of psychologists. The culture is one of biomedicine, which fosters power differences due to hierarchical relationships, a sense of personal responsibility for patient outcomes, an emphasis on clinical methods and experience, and often specialized, pragmatic thinking. The medical clinician's job is seen as that of finding an answer for and fixing the patient's problem. In other words, the primary goals are to cure disease and alleviate symptoms (Bray & Rogers, 1997). If these goals are unachievable, the goal then is to maintain or restore functioning. This is especially true for rural physicians who do not have ready access to specialists or colleagues to share responsibility for patient care.

Most physicians are trained in hospitals and have an extensive support staff. To navigate the primary care system, physicians learn the appropriate etiquette for practicing in medicosurgical hospitals and dealing with medical support staff. Decision making is vertically oriented with physicians having ultimate medicolegal responsibility for patient care.

In contrast, psychologists are trained in an array of theoretical positions that emphasize understanding and explanation derived from multiple theoretical models. Psychologists are trained to question everything, to gather and evaluate data, to generate provisional hypotheses, and to tolerate uncertainty and ambiguity in their work.

Physicians tend to be isolated from the laity in their professional culture, so they assume that everyone understands their culture and practices similarly. These cultural differences between medical practitioners and psychologists make communication and collaboration more difficult, unless these differences are understood and considered in practice.

Differences Between Medical Specialties

There are also unique training and cultural differences within the field of medicine (Bray & Rogers, 1997). In particular, generalists and primary care physicians are trained to look at the "big picture" (Donaldson, Yordy, & Vanselow, 1994) as they evaluate and care for patients. In particular, family physicians are trained to take care of their patients throughout the life cycle and to develop continuous, long-term relationships with their patients. This tendency is enhanced for rural physicians who often deliver children in the same family across several generations. Comprehensive care, easy accessibility, and unconditional acceptance of their patients are core attributes of primary care practitioners. From this vantage point, primary care practitioners may view psychologists like psychiatrists and other medical specialists in their care and relationship to patients.

Strategies for Success: Practice Styles and Issues

For psychologists to be successful they must understand medical culture and be prepared to respond creatively to the demands of this environment.

Psychologists and physicians have very different practice styles. For example, psychologists see about 1 patient per hour and 6 to 8 patients per day, whereas a busy physician sees 4 to 8 patients an hour and 40 to 60 patients per day. This practice pattern is changing for psychologists with pressures from managed care to see more patients in a shorter time period. Some psychologists are reporting seeing up to 2 patients in a 50-minute period (double the traditional 1 person per hour) because of extremely low managed-care reimbursement. Primary care physicians of necessity have short visits with patients, do brief intervention over multiple visits, and often consider giving a diagnosis to be a major part of the treatment (Bray & Rogers, 1997). This is particularly true for rural physicians who report seeing up to 80 patients per day simply because there is no other physician to share the workload.

The practical implications of these differences in practice styles are that the two professionals may have difficulty consulting with each other and may have different expectations about when and how patients are seen for diagnosis and treatment.

Confidentiality and Sharing Patient Records Between the Professions

Confidentiality and record sharing were two of the most difficult issues that arose in the Linkages Project, necessitating education, empathy, and mutual understanding. Physicians handle patient records differently from psychologists and are often not as protective of information. In many different settings, they talk readily to one another about cases, learning from one another, offering and receiving informal consultation and advice with little concern for the level of confidentiality demanded of a psychologist.

If psychologists are unable or unwilling to share information with primary care physicians about mutual patients, then working together is greatly impeded. Differences in expectations about confidentiality need to be resolved for successful collaboration to occur. It is usually the responsibility of the psychologist to clarify confidentiality issues with the patient and collaborating physician. To develop mutually respectful collaborative relationships, psychologists need to educate physicians about state confidentiality statutes and raise the level of consciousness of physicians about the devastating consequences of leaked information in the rural community. Once an understanding of the special protections afforded patients of psychologists is shared, communication becomes less problematic.

Stereotypes and Emotional Factors That Impede Collaborative Practice

Many psychologists have had both positive and negative experiences working with physicians (McDaniel et al., 1992) and consequently often express a considerable ambivalence about physicians. They may respect their work and physicians' position in the health care community on the one hand, while holding critical beliefs about "the medical model" on the other. In addition, professional socialization sometimes inculcates negative perceptions of physicians, because of psychologists' feelings of competition or their sense of belonging to a profession with less perceived overall power. If these attitudes are not changed both professionals suffer along with patient care. Psychologists need to develop successful collaborative relationships.

Linkage and Referrals

Physicians are trained in particular ways of making referrals. If psychologists do not understand and work to "fit" in with these expectations, they run the risk of being ignored. There are wide variations in these patterns. In general, physicians expect a contact after a referral is made to update them on the progress of the treatment. To facilitate information flow contact is often made with the office nurse or other support personnel in rural clinics.

There are also specific skills that physicians must have to make successful referrals: providing information that prepares patients and family members for collaborative care, preparing a patient and his or her family for a referral to a psychologist, including the psychologist in the evaluation of the referral, and clearly communicating expectations concerning the referral to the psychologist. The psychologist recipient of a referral can avoid a poor outcome by clarifying in each case what the referring physician's expectations are for the patient. Clearly, a hospital order written "psych consult stat" is not sufficient to this task.

Sophistication regarding the services provided by a psychologist varies greatly from physician to physician. The greatest potential for confusion between the professions has to do with the intention of the referring physician. To expedite the referral process, the psychologist should determine early whether the physician is referring the patient for on-going psychological care or is simply requesting a consultation. Once this determination has been made, the psychologist can ascertain the specific question that the physician wants to have answered from the consultation. This clarification is even more important in rural and frontier communities because people often have to travel great distances over difficult terrain to receive care.

Examples of consultation questions include differential diagnoses, specific recommendations for transfer or discharge planning, psychological co-morbidity affecting physical conditions, and iatrogenic effects of medication on the patient's well-being.

Financial Arrangements

Billing and payment arrangements can also be quite different in the two professions. Many physicians assume that psychologists will provide services to all of their patients and may not understand about practice limitations, such as psychologists not being Medicaid providers in certain states or not participating in a specific third-party or managed-care program. It is important to educate the physician regarding these limitations when establishing a collaborative relationship.

Methods for Developing Collaborative Practice

It is essential that there be regular and ongoing contact between the psychologist and primary care physician to maintain a good collaborative relationship. Methods that facilitate an ongoing relationship include having regular meetings or phone contacts, establishing referral routines, and clarifying referral and treatment expectations. In addition, it is necessary to work out collaborative relationships with support staff to ensure that important messages are conveyed in a timely manner. The person responsible for screening calls in the primary care physician's office is usually the office nurse. Successful collaboration can often be measured by the degree to which the office nurse recognizes the psychologist and assists in getting messages through to the physician.

Nontraditional Mental Health Practice

Collaborative practice may require the psychologist to break out of the traditional mode of seeing clients for 45 to 50 minutes of psychotherapy (Bray & Rogers, 1997). Alternative treatments and treatment formats, such as 15-minute consults, hospital consults, and hallway consults, are often necessary in these types of settings. A successful collaborative primary care physician–psychologist team often arranges to go on rounds together to make joint treatment plans and share observations, diagnostic assumptions, and concerns. Because there is virtually no public transportation available in rural areas collaborating psychologists and physicians have kept alive the time-honored tradition of the home visit.

Collaboration Factors

Several factors either facilitated or hindered collaboration between providers who participated in the Linkages Project. These factors can be readily extrapolated to rural practice (Bray & Rogers, 1995). Creating a specific collaboration plan was a key factor in the development of the working relationship. Professionals who had regular contact with each other were most likely to consult and to refer patients to each other. Practicing in close proximity also enhanced the linkage between providers. Participants who had regular meetings with each other or practiced in the same building were the most successful in establishing a collaborative relationship. Regular meetings included scheduled telephone contacts, lunch or breakfast appointments, use of faxes to make referrals, or contact during hospital rounds. Psychologists who made reciprocal referrals to physicians found much more receptive partners in their efforts. In many rural and frontier areas psychologists and physicians have created successful collaborations by office sharing. This is usually accomplished by having the psychologist visit the remote office of the physician on a rotating basis from once per week to once per month.

Small rural medicosurgical hospitals offer remarkable opportunities for collaboration for psychologists and primary health physicians. Observation of a young woman's brief stay in the primary care unit (PCU) of the community hospital in Jackson Hole, Wyoming, provides a great illustration. The patient was a 13-year-old girl hospitalized for a suicide attempt by a psychologist (psychologists have had privileges at this rural hospital) in collaboration with an obstetrician gynecologist primary care physician. The patient had recently become lethargic with episodes of agitation. Her moods were labile with rapid changes. During the agitation episodes she began cutting her forearms with a razor blade. She had, over the 2 days prior to admission, begun losing hair. Lab tests for thyroid dysfunction (T3, T4, and TSH) were normal. It was only when the physician suspected a rare form of Hypothyroidism (Wilson's disease) that follow up Free T3, TR tests (which measure thyroid hormone that is not attached to albumin) were ordered and the diagnosis confirmed. This young woman's response to thyroid supplement therapy was very dramatic. She went from Level 1 (lockdown) suicide precautions to discharge overnight. The physician's diagnostic skills and intervention were superb. The psychologist played a pivotal role working with the girl and her family during this dramatic emotional and psychological upheaval. This case illustrates the enhanced effectiveness of diagnosis and treatment consequent to collaboration in a rural community where professional roles are flexible and mutual respect exists between collaborating professionals.

Several factors can interfere with collaboration. Lack of proximity and regular settings for contact hindered referrals in the Linkages Project (Bray & Rogers, 1995). In many cases, psychologists may need to take the lead to develop the relationship and to establish a regular setting or routine for continuing the collaboration.

Managed-care and reimbursement issues are ongoing problems that interfere with collaborative practice. Not being on hospital staffs where physicians practice further interferes with collaboration. The hospital setting is a convenient place for informal and formal consultations between providers. Because many psychologists do not practice in general hospital settings, the opportunities for collaboration are decreased.

Conclusion

Given the continuing changes in the national health care system, psychologists will be required to modify their practice styles, and probably have greater opportunities to work closely with primary care physicians. Meeting the medical and mental health needs of patients necessitates the development of alternative models of service delivery, such as psychologists and physicians collaborating on prevention efforts and community health programs. To prepare for this new model of practice, psychologists need specific training in conceptualizing and implementing such collaborative efforts.

References

Bray, J. H., & Rogers, J. C. (1995). Linking psychologists and family physicians for collaborative practice. *Professional Psychology: Research and Practice, 26,* 132–138.

Bray, J. H., & Rogers, J. C. (1997). Training mental health professionals for collaborative practice with primary care physicians. *Families, Systems, & Health, 15,* 55–63.

Donaldson, M., Yordy, K., & Vanselow, N. (Eds.). (1994). *Defining primary care: An interim report* (Part 3). Committee on the Future of Primary Care, Division of Healthcare Services, Institute of Medicine (pp. 15–33). Washington, DC: National Academy Press.

Enright, M. F., & Blue, B. A. (1989). Collaborative treatment of panic disorders by psychologists and family physicians. *Psychotherapy in Private Practice, 7,* 85–90.

Enright, M. F., Resnick, R., DeLeon, P. H., Sciara, A. D., & Tanney, M. F. (1990). The practice of psychology in hospital settings. *American Psychologist, 45,* 1059–1065.

Glenn, M. L. (1985). Toward collaborative family-oriented health care. *Family Systems Medicine, 3,* 466–475.

Higgins, E. S. (1994). A review of unrecognized mental illness in primary care. *Archives of Family Medicine, 3,* 908–917.

Kroenke, K., & Mangelsdorff, D. (1989). Common symptoms in ambulatory care: Incidence, evaluation, therapy, and outcome. *American Journal of Medicine, 86,* 262–266.

McDaniel, S. H., Hepworth, J., & Doherty, W. J. (1992). *Medical family therapy.* New York: Basic Books.

Rakel, R. E. (1995). The family physician. In R. E. Rakel (Ed.), *Textbook of family practice* (5th ed., pp. 3–19). Philadelphia: W. B. Saunders.

5

Collaboration With Community Mental Health Centers

David S. Hargrove and Peter A. Keller

The diversity of health and mental health needs that is brought to professional service providers is staggering and requires an equally diverse workforce to respond effectively. In addition, the severity of the problems for which assistance is sought frequently demands not only that adequate providers be available but also that these persons work together in a competent and harmonious manner. Professional health care providers who work in primary care settings in rural communities must develop the skills to work cooperatively and collaboratively with persons from several other health and health-related disciplines.

Because rural communities do not usually have a wide array of mental health or medical service providers, particularly specialists, it is necessary that most serve as generalists (Hargrove, 1982). That is, they must be able to respond to a broad range of needs with a sufficient range of skills. Given the diversity of needs, it is unlikely that a small community of providers will have sufficient expertise to meet all needs. Thus, the configuration of providers, characterized by a network of psychologists, physicians, social workers, nurses, and other health and mental health service providers, must be responsive to the complex needs of persons and families in the community.

Collaborative relationships between health care and mental health providers are particularly important for several reasons. First, primary health care providers face an increasing number of patients who are experiencing mental health or psychological problems. A recent study of the lifetime and 12-month prevalence of psychiatric disorders found that nearly 50% of respondents described at least one lifetime disorder, whereas nearly 30% reported at least one 12-month disorder (Kessler et al., 1994). The prevalence of disorder is higher than had previously been assumed, and it is notable that a significant proportion of the individuals who reported a disorder had not obtained professional treatment.

Second, psychological components in physical illness are increasingly recognized as important factors in understanding and treating disease. In a managed-care environment, the cost-offset benefits of behavioral health care are increasingly being recognized in terms of their significance. Kelleher, Holmes, and Williams (1994) noted the increasing importance of consultation–liaison services and the rapid growth in the number of primary care clinicians practicing with associated services. An emphasis on treating the "whole patient" is gaining in prominence throughout health care systems for a variety of practical reasons.

Finally, the expectation that patients become active participants in their own care has taken hold in most health and mental health care systems. This expectation requires all health care providers to be more sensitive to the psychological needs of their patients if they are to provide responsive care. Each of these reasons underscores the importance of collaboration among health and mental health professionals who are involved in providing community services. The importance of this collaboration is even greater in rural communities where health care providers may be less accessible and less varied in discipline and specializations (Wagenfeld, Murray, Mohatt, & DeBruyn, 1994).

As psychologists become more involved in primary health care settings, it will be increasingly important to forge constructive relationships between health care organizations and community mental health centers (CMHCs). At this point it should be noted that there has been a growing diversity among CMHCs since the early 1980s, and they may take various forms depending on the state and community in which they are located. In some locales these agencies exist as free-standing and relatively comprehensive mental health centers; in others they may be agencies contracted to state or county government to provide mental health services; elsewhere the mental health provider may be a component of the county's human services program. These programs commonly employ a variety of professionals, including psychologists, psychiatrists, psychiatric social workers and nurses, and mental health counselors, and provide an array of mental health services. For consistency, we refer to CMHCs throughout this chapter.

Most CMHCs maintain rather large caseloads of seriously mentally ill persons and provide a broad range of outpatient, inpatient, and other treatment and rehabilitation services to persons experiencing a variety of mental health problems. Most also have in common pressures to maintain their services in the face of diminishing resources in a rapidly changing health care marketplace.

Despite the apparent value of collaborative work in health and mental health sectors, positive outcomes related to patient care are not always evident. Drotar (1993) made this clear in his comment,

> Despite testimony to the value of cooperative efforts, there is continuing evidence of a significant discrepancy between the promise and practice of collaboration ... Psychologists and physicians do not necessarily choose to work with one another, even when such collaboration may be helpful to clients. Collaborative opportunities in important clinical situations appear to be under exploited. (p. 160)

That we know so little about collaborative efforts is testimony to the lack of models for working together and to the forces that prevent interdisciplinary collaboration. Although we have found no data that pertain directly to rural settings, our observation is that rural communities may experience more informal collaboration because of the lower density of providers and the abovenoted tendency for practitioners to be more generalized in their practice.

This chapter identifies and addresses some of the issues pertaining to interdisciplinary collaboration, particularly staff members in community mental health settings and primary care providers. The hope is that it will provide assistance to providers as they develop skills to work cooperatively with persons from other professions on the health care team and, in turn, give better care to the consumers of both health and mental health services. In the first portion of the chapter we offer a brief description of human resource development in CMHCs and discuss more about the need for interdisciplinary collaboration. Afterward, we discuss some of the typical barriers to collaboration among providers. Finally, we offer suggestions for successful collaborative relationships.

Need for Collaboration

History of Collaboration

The changing face of health care in America is characterized by increased importance of the primary care setting for many aspects of health care delivery. This is particularly true in rural communities where people typically consult primary care providers for an increasingly broad range of both health and mental health needs. Consequently, community mental health centers must focus on primary care providers not merely as sources or objects of referrals, but as active partners in the delivery of comprehensive services. The relationship between community mental health programs and primary care providers must take the shape of an interdisciplinary effort as opposed to a multidisciplinary effort. Interdisciplinary work requires the meaningful interaction among providers who focus on a case in which multidisciplinary work merely brings all of the disciplines to the table with their varying perspectives. Rural communities demand that interdisciplinary, collaborative work be brought to bear on individual and family health and mental health issues (American Psychological Association Office of Rural Health, 1995).

Collaborative relationships, both within CMHC staff and outside with a variety of community agencies and health care practitioners, are an important aspect of the development of CMHCs. Typically, these are far more significant than mere resources for mutual referrals. The original 1963 federal legislation that created CMHCs stipulated that the staff of each center receiving federal funds must include a psychiatrist, psychologist, social worker, and nurse and recommended that persons of other disciplines involved with the rehabilitation of persons with mental illness also be involved. There was clear recognition of the value of multiple perspectives in the care and treatment of persons with mental illness. In addition to the variety of professional perspectives represented in the CMHC, centers were mandated to develop and maintain strong ties to the communities they were to serve. Virtually all centers had governing boards that were representative of the various components of the community. Advisory boards also provided input and offered opportunities for the development of collaborative relationships with a broader range of professionals and nonprofessionals. As family members and consumers began to play a more prominent role in the shaping of the health and mental health systems, they also assumed seats on governing and advisory boards for most publicly funded centers.

Emergence of Case Management

In the late 1970s and early 1980s, federal funding for community mental health centers yielded to block granting to states. Also, there emerged in public settings a new emphasis on serving seriously mentally ill adults and seriously emotionally disturbed children. Federal and state mental health authorities prioritized resources to serve those thought to be in the most need. Community support programs and child and adolescent service system projects were among the new initiatives introduced from the 1980s onward. With these changes there also emerged a heavy emphasis on case management for both children and adults. The new focus on case management typically prompted CMHCs to become more assertive in their efforts on behalf of the seriously mentally ill.

Although definitions of *case management* vary considerably, they typically involve one person who is responsible for ensuring the overall care and support services for a particular client. Frequently, case managers serve as advocates and brokers, enabling clients to gain access to the services and benefits needed for rehabilitation and recovery. Functionally, case managers became the representatives of the CMHC to the various professional health and mental health providers in a community. Because they operated on the boundary between the CMHC and other public and private providers in the community, the case managers ensured accessibility and availability of total community care for clients.

Whether the presence of case managers enhanced or sometimes impeded the development of collaborative relationships between local health and mental health providers and CMHC staffs has not been clearly demonstrated. It is clear, however, that case managers play a pivotal role in collaborative efforts to provide care because of their proximity and significance to clients, particularly those with serious mental illness. Many CMHCs assign their more highly trained staff —psychiatrists, psychologists, social workers, and psychiatric nurses—to directly billable activities and employ case managers mainly to arrange access to necessary support services and mental health and medical care.

As a result of the case management system, primary care professionals in a community, including psychologists in primary care settings, become involved with case managers from mental health centers. This typically occurs even prior to involvement with the treating professionals who work in the same CMHCs. Although communication about patients frequently flows through case managers, it typically is necessary for providers involved in active treatment with patients also to maintain clear and open channels for information and dialogue.

Because persons with serious mental illness are vulnerable

to physical illness, dental problems, homelessness, difficulties sustaining employment, and problems gaining access to social support resources, effective interdisciplinary teams are important to the well-being of these people and their families. Sometimes the teams are sustained through the work of case managers; other times they must rely on the communication and negotiation skills of the providers who are working directly with the patients. In rural areas that are characterized by a limited number of providers and facilities, it is likely that CMHC staff and other local providers will be mutually involved with a large number of patients and families, enabling them to forge complementary roles and expectations through experience.

Barriers to Collaboration

There are many barriers that prevent professional health and mental health service providers from working collaboratively. These barriers can be conceptualized as structural or personal. Structural barriers consist of characteristics of institutions or systems of care that impede collaborative work between persons of different disciplines. Personal barriers consist of characteristics of the persons or groups of professional persons that prevent collaborative work. These categories are purely conceptual and should not necessarily be regarded as discrete, but simply as convenient ways of organizing thinking about barriers to collaboration. For example, it is not always clear whether the rationale for refusal to collaborate with another person or profession is due to the institution for which one works or because of one's personal experiences or preferences.

Structural Barriers. Structural barriers to collaboration include external forces that prohibit or prevent successful cooperative work between health and mental health providers. They may be rooted in institutions, professional associations, accreditation, training models, or political and business agreements. Examples of structural barriers include institutionally determined hierarchies of power relationships, well-established cultures of relationships between professions or disciplines, recognition of certain groups as privileged and others as not privileged, and the inclusion of certain individuals and exclusion of others in decision-making processes. For example, certain aspects of traditional medical settings are clearly hierarchical, and such structures may clash with the need to collaborate. Structural barriers also may be described in terms of the environment in which collaboration occurs. Lowe and Herranen (1981) developed a model of multidisciplinary teamwork that is based on an environment that allows the concept of teamwork to be understood and practiced. Their model is based on a belief in the equal value of each participant on the team and the shared values of "open communication, shared leadership, decision-making and responsibility" (p. 4).

Personal Barriers. Personal barriers to collaboration are those internal characteristics of significant "players" within institutions and organizations where collaboration is a possibility. These include attitudes, beliefs, expectations, idiosyncratic motives, and perspectives that may either be assets or impediments to harmonious working relationships with other agencies or organizations. Examples of personal barriers would be one professional person's belief that he or she should always be the team leader or final decision maker regardless of the task or nature of the group, or an opinion by one person or group that a particular discipline is preeminent in the care of patients, or the expectation that one person must exclusively determine the nature of assessment and treatment planning for clients of an agency.

Koeske, Koeske, and Mallinger (1993) identified another example of personal barriers. They studied perceptions of professional competence among psychologists, social workers, and psychiatrists and found, not surprisingly, that each group was biased toward itself in terms of helpfulness, expertise, warmth, and as the preferred recipient of referrals. Although the authors did not study whether these perceptions limited the willingness or tendency to collaborate, it may be presumed that these perceptions offer the basis for attitudes that would influence the willingness and ability to collaborate.

The strength of the professional identities of the collaborators also is a variable that may be either a barrier or contributor to a collaborative effort. Erikson (1950) noted that one's capacity for reciprocal relationships was rooted in his or her personal identity. In the professional context, the caregiver with a well-developed professional identity, based on confidence not requiring defensiveness, is more likely to be able to work in a mutually supportive, reciprocal relationship with others. On the basis of this thinking, it seems more likely that a person with a well-developed professional identity would also be able to respect another, similar group.

It seems unlikely that one's professional identity will develop in a healthy, nondefensive manner unless there are persons of other professions in the same training or practice context. Without this experience and opportunity for comparison, there is little opportunity to forge one's own thinking and development about professional matters. It frequently has been pointed out that few if any health or mental health professional persons have training experiences in collaborative activity and that interdisciplinary work is relatively rare until quite late in most training programs, if it occurs at all. It is not at all unusual for community mental health professionals to have their first interdisciplinary collaborative experiences after they have been employed. Background information concerning these and related issues is provided in a recent monograph that outlines an interdisciplinary curriculum for mental health providers working in rural settings (American Psychological Association Office of Rural Health, 1995).

There certainly are formidable structural and personal barriers to collaboration. In the face of these barriers, however, are the forces that stress the practice of collaborative skills among mental health professionals who wish to work in a health care environment. There are several reasons for these collaborative skills. First, the sheer diversity of health and mental health problems that demand response require multiple perspectives. Second, the complexity of the social systems in which rehabilitation and recovery occur necessitates several types of professional expertise, ranging from clinical skills to community organization. Third, the interaction of diverse problems with complex rehabilitation systems requires a dynamic collaborative interchange between professionals who are focusing on the same case. This type of collaborative activity assures that professional persons will focus on the many dimensions of mental health needs of a given consumer while working in a multifaceted context. It is not at all likely that one profession can provide an adequate perspective to embrace the multiple needs of any given client population, particularly those persons with serious mental illness. Thus, the collaborative work of several professionals within a specified context is most likely to be of greatest benefit to clients and other consumers of services.

Although not conceptualized as barriers, Drotar (1993) described three sets of influences on collaborative outcomes. They include the following: "(a) participants' beliefs about the need for and expectations of collaborative outcomes; (b) participants' knowledge, skills, and prior experience in collaborative activities; and (c) setting-based barriers and supports" (p. 164). Presumably, each needs to be explored for successful collaboration to occur.

Suggestions for Collaboration

Although there still is little evidence of successful collaboration, particularly between psychologists and physicians, there continues to be optimism among some health and mental health service providers that reciprocal, collaborative relationships will work. Serious thinking and efforts to establish collaborative programs are beginning to emerge (Bray, Enright, & Rogers, this volume; Morris, this volume). Drotar, a pediatric psychologist, provides a useful model for collaboration among professionals that serves as a guide for collaborative activities as well as an heuristic guide for research and evaluation of such activities. His model is based on the relationships between pediatricians and pediatric psychologists and offers a structure by which other collaborative relationships can be conceptualized.

Drotar's (1993) model is based on his definition of *interdisciplinary collaboration*:

> At the broadest level, interdisciplinary collaboration can be defined as any professional activity that is conducted between a member of one profession and another. Collaboration occurs between individuals, which is how we typically think of it, at a program level, that is, among groups of psychologists and pediatricians in a particular setting, or in professional organizations. The goals and content of collaborative activities are heterogeneous. (p. 161)

Although his thinking developed in the pediatric context, the definition and model of *interdisciplinary collaboration* can be extended to other health and mental health professions from various institutional settings who seek to collaborate.

Drotar (1993) identified several components of collaboration to define his model. These components include dimensions of collaborative activity and influences of collaborative activity. The dimensions of collaboration include the goals and content, types of settings, characteristics of participants, variables in the relationship between the participants, and the outcomes.

Examples of goals and content of the collaboration may include teaching, clinical care, case management, research, program administration, program evaluation, and professional organization. Types of settings may include a CMHC, an independent practice of medicine or psychology, a medicosurgical hospital, a private psychiatric hospital, or a state psychiatric hospital. Characteristics of the participants may include how many are involved, their discipline or professional identification, training and experience, and previous relationships. Relationship variables include its history and duration, frequency of contact, type of contact, and authority and control. Outcomes may include referrals, economic gain, improved care and service development, new knowledge, grants, publications, and professional satisfaction.

In his discussion of influences on collaborative activity,

Drotar (1993) pointed out the importance of the stage of the collaboration. For example, in a long-term collaborative relationship, the initial phase will focus on quite different issues than a more immediate and time-limited collaboration. The first phase of the long-term collaboration will no doubt focus on such concerns as structure, membership, purpose, and outcomes. As the relationship matures, these issues will be dealt with according to the mores that have developed within the relationship. In more focused, short-term collaborative activities, however, the task itself dominates the structure and activity of the group. Specific issues of patient care or the development of a prescribed program are examples of outcomes that may result from short-term collaboration.

Drotar (1993) focused considerable attention on the specific influences on the outcomes of collaboration. They include beliefs and expectations, skills, and situational incentives and constraints. Beliefs and expectations include confidence that the collaboration is necessary and effective, and specific beliefs that participants may have about role and authority issues within collaborative relationships. Examples of important skills include problem identification, effective utilization of information, and communication and interpersonal skills. Situational incentives and constraints include accessibility, time pressures, multiple responsibilities, funding patterns, reimbursement patterns, and administrative organization.

Specific outcomes of the collaboration activity may include reciprocal use of services by several disciplines, joint research and training, and mutually beneficial consultation. Consequences of these outcomes may include perceived benefits and satisfaction by participants, more efficient and effective patient care, economic benefits, and results that are specific to one or more of the institutions (e.g., publications or credibility in the community).

Although Drotar's (1993) model has not been extensively evaluated, it offers a plausible sequence of components, relationships, and processes that can guide collaborative activity. Its use can provide some order in the collaborative process, enhancing the possibilities of success and certainly making easier more precise evaluation.

Conclusion

Rural settings present a special circumstance wherein collaborative relationships between psychologists and other health service providers hold great potential for improving the quality of all services. Interdisciplinary collaboration between health and mental health providers and community mental health programs presumably will enhance the outcomes of clinical care as well as increase job satisfaction among caregivers. Although there is little empirical validation of the impact of interdisciplinary collaboration, there continues to be optimism about its influence on health and mental health practice, particularly in rural areas where there are limited human resources. The identification of a specific model, such as Drotar's (1993), increases the possibilities of validating and improving the processes of collaboration. Regardless of the specific model of collaborative work, it is clear that attention must be paid to the process of collaboration. Evaluations of these relationships should involve both the outcomes of the interdisciplinary relationships and the processes that were involved to reach them. Providing the perspective of evaluation as well as the methodologies by which evaluation will take place is an important contribution that the psychologist can make to the interdisciplinary team that involves primary care providers and mental health center professionals.

References

American Psychological Association Office of Rural Health. (1995). *Caring for the rural community: An interdisciplinary curriculum.* Washington, DC: American Psychological Association.

Drotar, D. (1993). Influences on collaborative activities among psychologists and pediatricians: Implications for practice, training, and research. *Journal of Pediatric Psychology, 18,* 159–172.

Erikson, E. (1950). *Childhood and society.* New York: Norton.

Hargrove, D. S. (1982). The rural psychologist as generalist: A challenge for professional identity. *Professional Psychology, 13,* 302–308.

Kelleher, K., Holmes, T. M., & Williams, C. (1994). *Major recent trends in mental health in primary care.* (DHHS Pub. No. SMA 943000). Washington, DC: U.S. Government Printing Office.

Kessler, R. C., McGonagle, K. A., Zhao, S., Nelson, C. B., Hughes, M., Eshleman, S., Wittchen, H., & Kendler, K. S. (1994). Lifetime and 12-month prevalence of *DSM-III-R* psychiatric disorders in the United States. *Archives of General Psychiatry, 51,* 8–19.

Koeske, G. F., Koeske, R. D., & Mallinger, J. (1993). Perceptions of professional competence: Cross-disciplinary ratings of psychologists, social workers, and psychiatrists. *American Journal of Orthopsychiatry, 63,* 45–54.

Lowe, J. I., & Herranen, M. (1981). Understanding teamwork: Another look at basic concepts. *Social Work in Healthcare, 7,* 1–11.

Wagenfeld, M. O., Murray, J. D., Mohatt, D. F., & DeBruyn, J. C. (1994). *Mental health and rural America: 1980–1993* (NIH Publication No. 94-3500). Washington, DC: U.S. Department of Health and Human Services.

6

The Rural Psychologist in the Hospital Emergency Room

Jerry A. Morris

The rural medicosurgical hospital emergency room (ER) is the safety net of the rural community. It is the place where worried parents bring children during the night for assessment, treatment, and reassurance; where loved ones with chest pains are evaluated and treated; where patients are stabilized; and where bewildered posttransient ischemic attack seniors are treated.

Psychologists have had hospital privileges in some states since the late 1970s (Enright, Resnick, Ludwigsen, & DeLeon, 1993). Rural psychologists have contributed as practitioners to community health centers since the mid-1960s (Bennett et al., 1966). By 1982 10% of psychologists worked primarily in hospitals (Manderscheid & Sonnenschein, 1991). To assist them with hospital practice during the mid-1980s, the American Psychological Association (APA) published *A Hospital Practice Primer for Psychologists* (1985), which outlined credentialing, bylaws requirements, standards, and procedures for psychologists practicing in hospitals. In 1985 the Joint Commission on Accreditation of Healthcare Organizations (JCAHO) published standards that allowed hospitals to include nonphysician providers on hospital staffs (Enright et al., 1993).

Psychologist–Physician Collaboration

The rural hospital ER is traditionally the facility of first resort for people seeking assistance with a myriad of physical and behavioral health problems. The majority of patients with mental illness are seen in primary care centers (Brody, 1996; Regier, Goldberg, & Taube, 1978; Schulberg & Scott, 1991). Unlike urban centers, specialized care institutions are often unavailable, or are accessible only at great distances. Emergency care may require local hospital stabilization, assessment, and later transport to a distant facility should prolonged inpatient mental health treatment become necessary. These needs are likely to continue and even expand under privatization of mental health services in a managed-care environment (White, Bateman, Fisher, & Geller, 1995). Primary care centers have increasingly become the gatekeepers for more specialized services, such as mental health and substance abuse treatment (Narrow et al., 1993). This shift to comprehensive screening and service facilitation in the rural ER will usher in an era in which multidisciplinary staffing and team work will be essential.

The rural physician covering the ER often depends on the rural psychologist to assist with the emergency assessment of patients needing evaluation, and to link up with mental health facilities for placement when transfer is required. The psychologist depends on the physician for the physical screening of patients admitted to the general hospital for brief stabilization of depression and anxiety disorders, and for evaluation of patients for pharmacological interventions. The physician counts on the psychologist to meet with the families of hospitalized patients, to interface with schools and juvenile officers, to arrange medical leaves of absence with employers, and to identify and interface with outpatient services that can provide aftercare.

The psychologist provides lab results: historical data, psychological assessment; testing; and extensive clinical interviews of individual, family, and significant others. This essential information improves the accuracy and relevance of the treatment team's diagnosis and justifies the hospital stay.

The rural psychologist often has intimate knowledge of the patient and the patient's family prior to presentation in the ER. The psychologist and physician collaborate to make a comprehensive assessment and to initiate appropriate treatment. They jointly lead a team of professionals (nurses, hospital social workers, insurance case managers, outpatient practitioners, and involved state and federal agencies) to establish patient engagement in the therapy process and to plan the aftercare linkage. This teamwork distributes responsibility and minimizes patient resistance and complaints.

This collaboration among the ER staff, general hospital physician, and psychologist has become a meaningful component in many training programs and has resulted in collaborative efforts on the part of APA and the American Academy of Family Practice Physicians. Bray and Rogers (1995) chronicled the collaborative efforts and recent affiliation of these two professional associations and the APA Rural Health Task Force. Participants in the psychologist–physician collaboration pairs focusing on alcohol and other substance abuse indicated that the program was successful in improving the level and quality of collaborative practice and that the collaboration resulted in enhanced effectiveness of each professional in diagnosing and treating medical and psychosocial problems (Bray & Rogers, 1995).

For collaboration to work, effective institutional leadership committed to clearly identified institutional goals must exist. This leadership must be flexible, innovative, and sensitive to the needs of the practitioners involved (Yank et al., 1991). Leaders (board members, administrators, chiefs of medical staff, chiefs of psychology services, and directors of nursing) should be role models who are willing to commit the resources and personal time to ensure that collaborative efforts are effective.

Setting Specific Variables

Emerging models stress the integration of primary care centers and psychological services to respond to the prevalence of psychological and behavioral problems in society, and to the increasing incidence of these problems encountered in the typical ER (Morris, 1995a). The best estimates of prevalence indicate that approximately 10 individuals in 100 in the United States suffer from mental disorder (Kaplan & Sadock, 1985; Regier et al., 1984). When one considers that the prevalence of alcohol and drug abuse or dependence can run as high as another 20 patients per 100 individuals in the general population (Regier et al., 1984, Regier et al., 1990), the ER screening problem starts to come into focus. It has been determined that as much as 57% of all citizens will suffer from a mental disorder in their lifetime, with 20% requiring psychological intervention (Regier et al., 1984). The prevalence of serious and persistent mental illness during any 12-month period is estimated to be 3.3 million adults 18 years of age or older, with as many as 18.2 adults per 1,000 within any year being so severely disabled by psychological disorders that they warrant classification as chronically mentally ill (Barker et al., 1989).

Approximately 1 in 7 to 1 in 4 individuals being screened in a hospital ER will have a diagnosable substance abuse, psychological problem, or both (Morris, 1995a). Many researchers maintain that there are generally no consistent urban–rural differences in the prevalence of such diagnostic groups as affective disorders, anxiety disorders, somatization disorders, alcohol abuse, cognitive impairments, and antisocial personality (Robins & Regier, 1990). However, rural residents are less likely than urban residents to receive specialty care for psychological problems, and whereas 28% of the nation's population live in rural communities, less than 0.1% of the psychiatric hospital beds are there, and 61% of the rural population live in a designated psychiatric–psychological personnel shortage area (National Institute of Mental Health, 1978; National Rural Health Association, 1993, p. 22; Redick, 1976). Others indicate that rural citizens experience increased prevalence of alcohol abuse, child and spouse abuse, and depression (Hargrove & Breazeale, 1993; National Mental Health Association, 1988).

Regardless of the comparison of rural to urban prevalence rates, the clinical needs of the rural individual are significant

(Beeson & Johnson, 1987; Garfinkel, Hoberman, Parsons, & Walker, 1990; Heffernan & Heffernan, 1987; Rosenberg, 1986). Unlike the urban centers with multiple hospitals in close proximity, specialized psychiatric hospitals and day treatment facilities available minutes away, and a broad array of doctors of psychology and psychiatry available, rural hospitals often must rely on collaboration between a handful of general physicians and one or two psychologists or a part-time consulting psychiatrist who lives in a remote urban center.

The difficulty with access to psychological services may result from many rural hospitals not having traditionally integrated psychologists and other professionals on ER staffs and regular on-call rotations, or because psychosocial problems are given a low priority by the facility and by house physicians (Schuster, 1995). However, other variables are worthy of consideration. Primary care physicians have a poor track record of detecting, accurately diagnosing, and appropriately treating or referring mental health and substance abuse problems (Beeson, 1994; Houpt, Orleans, George, & Brodie, 1979; Morris, 1994; Morris, 1995b; Muszynski, Brady, & Sharfstein, 1987; Parlour, Young, Jones, & Brady, 1985; Smith, 1993). In fact, the recognition rate of mental disorders by primary care physicians in hospital settings has been surveyed at from 10% to 50% (Nielsen & Williams, 1980; Schulberg, Saul, McClelland, et al., 1985).

Medical specialists in ER care have admitted that medical staff members are often unprepared for screening and treating the psychologically disturbed patient (Borges, Summers, & Karshmer, 1995). Less than 1% of acute care medical patients have been reported to receive psychological care and treatment for their mental health symptoms (Shahinpour, Hollinger-Smith, & Perlia, 1995).

Many rural hospital administrators are worried about low hospital census rates. Board members are concerned about the long-term survivability of rural hospitals. As managed-care and systems contracting approaches permeate the health care delivery system, medical staff members are increasingly concerned about the quality and comprehensiveness of care and of case management in rural hospitals. Many of these leaders will consider using psychologists to refer patients, maintain on-call availability for unattached house cases, screen accurately and appropriately and triage patients, and establish ER physician–psychologist teams (Morris, 1995a).

The Psychologist's ER Functions

The psychologist collaborating with physicians in the ER will need strong evaluation and diagnostic skills, multidisciplinary team experience, structural and procedural support, and a serious commitment both to the hospital professional staff and to patients' continuous and emergent needs.

The ER staff role demands 24-hour, daily responsibilities. Participation in the rural hospital ER requires that the psychologist practice with professional responsibility, shared liability, dependability, and integrity achievable only in a hospital setting in which the commitment, training, and skills of the psychologist are openly appreciated, acknowledged, and reinforced.

The Evaluation

The general physician has usually completed a medical screening and identified one or more psychological symptoms or components of the patient's presenting problem before the psychologist is involved in the case. Many efficient ER staffs adopt one or more brief screening devices, which the intake nursing staff can administer during the process of getting initial information. Short checklists are often used because of their brevity and ease of application.

As the physician identifies psychological symptoms he or she usually explains to the patient that a doctor specializing in psychological problems is a part of the ER team and that he or she will be asking that doctor to participate in the comprehensive assessment of the patient's problems. Most general hospital ERs provide a posted list of rotating on-call psychologists and psychiatrists or allow the attending physician to bypass the list and call in the practitioner of his or her preference.

The physician will either ask the nurse to call the psychologist for immediate consultation or determine that the patient needs hospital admission for further treatment and work-up (diagnostic and laboratory assessment). The physician will ask the nurse to notify the psychologist that the patient is being admitted and will require an assessment and work-up within the next 24 hours. When called in on an ER consultation, the psychologist must respond immediately. In the rural medicosurgical hospital this situation occurs an average two to three times per week.

The necessity for immediate response requires that the rural hospital psychologist have an office near the hospital or in the medical complex. Many rural physicians and psychologists select offices adjacent to the hospital or arrange to lease office space in the hospital complex's medical arts building. Certainly, the carrying of a paging system or beeper is a must for the rural hospital psychologist, as after hours on-call access is just as important to the ER as office hour access. Many rural hospital psychologists, like rural physicians, take one or more partners so that the on-call responsibility can be shared. This allows the doctor of psychology with ER responsibilities to take time off and assures the hospital that there is backup available during vacations, sickness, and family emergencies.

The significant point is that ER psychologists must be available on a moment's notice. If they are seeing an office patient during an ER call, they must inform the patient and the ER about the length of time it will take to get to the ER, when they will return, and whether their outpatient should wait or reschedule. (This situation creates ethical concerns about the "breach" of a patient's session of psychotherapy; monetary loss due to interrupted sessions that cannot be filled; and the stress on the patient and doctor.) These actions take coordination and experience. Appropriately prepared, most outpatients appreciate the commitment of the doctor who will see them in the ER during a crisis and are surprisingly understanding and flexible when they must wait for their outpatient session, have the session cut short, or have to reschedule.

Hospital administrators and staff must realize that, for the psychologist to cover emergent situations in the ER, he or she makes considerable sacrifice and manages significant levels of stress. He or she also makes financial sacrifices such as contracting for close proximity office space, losing some patients who don't feel that they can adjust to interrupted or delayed outpatient sessions, and making the commitment to follow patients seen in the ER if other practitioners are not available, thus filling up available practice hours that might be more efficiently allocated to higher paying consulting work. Additional layers of professional responsibility and stress and the loss of some personal lifestyle freedom are other costs related to ER work.

Once involved in an ER case, the psychologist is best advised to introduce himself or herself as a member of the multidisciplinary team that is attending to the emergent problem. In this manner, he or she establishes a collaborative frame that often allays the patient's anxiety about being evaluated for a psychological condition (Schuster, 1995). Generally, it is good to alert the patient to hospital procedures and rules that require that a specialist assess certain problems during ER episodes and in this way communicate that the procedure of psychological evaluation is reasonably routine. This approach often helps the patient experience the process as less personally intrusive and pejorative.

The first 15 minutes of the usual ER psychological evaluation are dedicated to the compilation of a "brief history." This includes a focused interview with the patient and significant others who are available to establish a psychological database that includes significant information related to the admission and the determination of personal, familial, and professional resources available for aftercare.

The psychologist will efficiently compile information concerning the patient's chief complaint and the circumstances leading up to ER admission; the patient's past treatment history and the effect of specific interventions; the family's history of mental illness; the patient's and family's substance abuse patterns and history; the patient's occupational, educational, and legal status; the history of violence or aggression toward self and others; recent losses; pattern of interaction in significant relationships; personal philosophy and belief system; current professionals considered active treaters; and historical capacity to be engaged in the treatment process. The skilled ER psychologist can actually cover a great deal of ground with an individual in an acute phase of a psychological illness in a very short time. This experience and skill add significantly to the depth and utility of the ER assessment.

The second 15 minutes of the ER psychological evaluation are usually spent in a standard mental status examination (MSE). During the MSE, the psychologist reviews systems of functioning, establishing level of reality orientation; intellectual level, abstracting ability, and indicators of cognitive functioning; level of insight and judgment; mood and general affect management skills; ego strength; identity formation and level of socialization; defensive style and ability to manage impulses; current suicidal or homicidal ideation or plans or dangerousness to self and others; central nervous system deficits; capacity for bonding and availability in interpersonal relationships; and the level of rationality of plans for addressing the current problem.

By the end of the first half hour with the patient, the ER psychologist generally has significant historical and interactive data on which to base a tentative diagnosis and to formulate an initial treatment plan. This database has often been tested against the information and impressions of available significant others accompanying the patient or over the telephone. Often, because of the nature of the rural treatment community, the ER psychologist has access to additional data from previous treatment experience with the patient, past psychological testing, or telephone communication with local practitioners currently treating the patient.

In this fashion, the multidisciplinary ER team that includes the psychologist amasses a wealth of psychological data to correlate with physical and nursing assessment. ER staffs organized in this fashion are well prepared to ensure accurate diagnosis, comprehensive treatment planning, coordination with ancillary and supportive resources, and the safety of the patient and community.

Disposition and Treatment

Once comprehensive evaluation is completed, the multidisciplinary team operating in the hospital ER must make important decisions relative to patient placement, treatment and the time of onset of intervention, and linkage with aftercare services. Generally, these decisions start with consideration of current dangerousness, the patient's current capacity and willingness to assume some responsibility for caring for himself or herself, the seriousness of the diagnosis, the patient's and family's historical pattern of response, and the availability and accessibility of treatment resources. The psychologist's evaluation positions the treatment team to make these decisions.

On the basis of the evaluation of these variables, the team can decide on (and document the need for) immediate hospitalization (voluntary or involuntary). The team can choose ER intervention with crisis psychotherapy followed by coordination with outpatient facilities or practitioners and consideration for pharmacological intervention, or consultation and discharge with recommendations. In this manner, there is a body of knowledge gathered in a comprehensive and standardized fashion that meets the community standards of care. Such a database used in a thoughtful and professional manner, to reach a reasonable clinical conclusion, is invaluable to the patient and team when crisis situations emerge. This format ensures quality, extends the attending physician's and hospital's liability to the psychologist expert, and demonstrates linkage and coordination of care when hospital admission is not effected.

An additional benefit of this approach to ER assessment and treatment using a psychologist member of the team is a closer relationship with referral sources. In the rural community, the hospital is dependent on a wide variety of referral sources to maintain the census necessary for continued existence. This model ensures that ER-assessed patients suffering from mental disorder get linked with community resources. Although community mental health practitioners are consequently valued, are aided by referrals, and are linked effectively to the hospital, the hospital in return increases its utilization rates and census, and enhances its image as a comprehensive health care center.

Accountability and Cost-Effectiveness

In the emerging era of managed health care services and performance contracting, hospitals will be hard pressed to document thoroughly the need for admission, demonstrate that active interventions for all diagnoses are available, and demonstrate that reasonable lengths of stay with linkage with appropriate outpatient aftercare are components of hospital interventions. Psychological services have demonstrated effectiveness, and often reduce annual health care expenditures (Cummings, Dorken, Pallak, & Henke, 1990; Morris, 1995a). In fact, psychological interventions have demonstrated that, when they are used in combination with medications, 1-year relapse rates are cut in half (Hogarty et al., 1991). Psychological treatment strategies, used in combination with medications, produce reduction of target symptoms, improved social functioning, and lower relapse rates (Bellack, Turner, Hersen, & Luber, 1984; Eckman et al., 1992; Hogarty et al., 1986; Hogarty et al., 1991; Paul & Lentz, 1977; Wallace & Liberman, 1985).

Evidence is mounting that the more psychotherapy and related services patients in some treatment populations receive, the better the outcome (Baker, Jodrey, Intagliatia, & Straus, 1993; Durell, Lechtenberg, Corse, & Frances, 1993; McLellan, Arndt, Metzger, Woody, & O'Brien, 1993). Data are even available that indicate that the coordinated multidisciplinary team and case-management approach outlined above are both treatment effective and cost-effective (Baker et al., 1993; Durrell et al., 1993; McLellan et al., 1993; Morris, 1995a).

Research findings clarify the cost and outcome effectiveness of psychotherapy and psychological services. Multidisciplinary teams that deliver coordinated and case-managed services are also establishing outcome effectiveness. The ER seeking to establish credibility with managed patient systems will increasingly seek the services of psychologists, use multidisciplinary teams, and demonstrate linkage with outpatient psychological services.

Conclusion

The significant prevalence of psychological disorders in patients seeking evaluation and treatment in ERs and the comprehensive diagnostic and intervention skills of the clinical psychologist provide an opportunity for rural hospitals to positively affect the quality of diagnosis and treatment in emergency service centers. Powerful psychological evaluation tools and procedures constitute an important addition to the experience and talent of the general physician and nurse. These psychological skills include interdisciplinary team leadership, accessibility and availability, focused and parsimonious evaluation of the patient's clinical needs, linkage and collaboration with community resources, availability for ongoing outpatient care of the patient, and proven cost and treatment effectiveness of psychological interventions.

The ER psychologist provides the rural hospital with the opportunity to limit liability. The psychologist can also assist the hospital with demonstrating to supervising agencies that comprehensive determination of need or lack of need for hospitalization and linkage with appropriate outpatient services have been accomplished. The psychologist can assist the hospital with establishing closer ties to the community mental health practitioners who can act as significant referral sources.

The rural hospital administrator, board member, and staff physician seeking to improve the quality of ER services, enhance the hospital's image and effectiveness, and strengthen documentation and compliance with standards of care will increasingly include psychologists on ER staffs and on-call rotations. The psychologist and physician make an especially powerful team in the rural health care environment.

References

American Psychological Association. (1985). *A hospital practice primer for psychologists.* Washington, DC: Author.

Baker, F., Jodrey, D., Intagliatia, J., & Straus, H. (1993). Community support services and functioning of the seriously mentally ill. *Community Mental Health Journal, 29,* 321–331.

Barker, P., Manderscheid, R., Hendershot, G., Jack, S., Schoenborn, C., & Goldstrom, I. (1989). Serious mental disability in the adult household population: United States, 1989. In R. Manderscheid & M. Sonnerschein (Eds.), *Mental health, United States, 1992* (pp. 255–268). Washington, DC: U.S. Government Printing Office.

Beeson, P. G. (1994). The state mental health/substance abuse perspective. In J. A. Merchant, R. Ungar, & D. McMillan (Eds.), *Implementing healthcare reform in rural America: State and community roles* (pp. 351–371). Iowa City, IA: University of Iowa Press.

Beeson, P. G., & Johnson, D. R. (1987, May). *A panel study of changes (1981–86) in rural mental health status: Effects of the rural crisis.* Paper presented at the National Institute of Mental Health National Conference on Mental Health Statistics, Denver, CO.

Bellack, A. S., Turner, S. M., Hersen, M., & Luber, R. F. (1984). An examination of the efficacy of social skills training for chronic schizophrenic patients. *Hospital and Community Psychiatry, 35,* 1023–1028.

Bennett, C. C., Anderson, L. S., Cooper, S., Hassol, L., Klein, D. C., & Rosenblum, G. (Eds.). (1966). *Community psychology: A report of the Boston Conference on the Education for Psychologists in Community Mental Health.* Boston: Boston University Press.

Borges, W. J., Summers, L. C., & Karshmer, J. (1995). Psychiatric emergency service. Using available resources. *Journal of Nursing Administration, 25,* 31–37.

Bray, J. H., & Rogers, J. C. (1995). Linking psychologists and family physicians for collaborative practice. *Professional Psychology: Research and Practice, 26,* 132–133.

Brody, D. S. (1996). What is the role of the primary care physician in managed mental health care? In A. Lazarus (Ed.), *Controversies in managed mental health care* (pp. 29–40). Washington, DC: American Psychiatric Press.

Cummings, N. A., Dorken, H., Pallak, M. S., & Henke, C. (1990). *The impact of psychological intervention on healthcare utilization and costs: The Hawaii Medicaid Project* (Report No. 11-C-98344/9). San Francisco: Biodyne Institute.

Durell, J., Lechtenberg, B., Corse, S., & Frances, R. (1993). Alcohol and drug abuse: Intensive case management of persons with chronic mental illness who abuse substances. *Hospital and Community Psychiatry, 44,* 415–416, 428.

Eckman, T. A., Wirshing, W. C., Marder, S. R., Liberman, R. P., Johnston-Cronk, K., Zimmerman, K., & Mintz, J. (1992). Technique for training schizophrenic patients in illness self-management: A controlled trial. *American Journal of Psychiatry, 149,* 1549–1555.

Enright, M. F., Resnick, R. J., Ludwigsen, K. R., & DeLeon, P. H. (1993). Hospital practice: Psychology's call to action. *Professional Psychology: Research and Practice, 24,* 135–141.

Garfinkel, B. D., Hoberman, H., Parsons, J., & Walker, J. (1990). *The prevalence of depression and suicide attempts in rural Minnesota youth: A preliminary report.* In M. O. Wagenfeld, J. D. Murray, D. F. Mohatt, & J. C. DeBruyn (Eds.), *Mental health and rural America: 1980–1993.* Rockville, MD: National Institute of Mental Health.

Hargrove, D. S., & Breazeale, R. L. (1993). Psychologists and rural services: Addressing a new agenda. *Professional Psychology: Research and Practice, 24,* 319–324.

Heffernan, W. D., & Heffernan, J. B. (1987). *Testimony prepared for a hearing of the Joint Economic Committee of the Congress of the United States.* (Available from W. D. Heffernan, Department of Rural Sociology, University of Missouri, Columbia, MO 65201.)

Hogarty, G. E., Anderson, C. M., Reiss, D. J., Kornblith, S. J., Greenwald, D. P., Javna, C. D., & Madonia, M. J. (1986). Family psychoeducation, social skills training, and maintenance chemotherapy in the aftercare treatment of schizophrenia: I. One-year effects of a controlled study on relapse and expressed emotion. *Archives of General Psychiatry, 43,* 633–642.

Hogarty, G. E., Anderson, C. M., Reiss, D. J., Kornblith, S. J., Greenwald, D. P., Ulrich, R. F., & Carter, M. (1991). Family psychoeducation, social skills training, and maintenance chemotherapy in the aftercare treatment of schizophrenia: II. Two year effects of a controlled study on relapse and adjustment. *Archives of General Psychiatry, 48,* 340–347.

Houpt, J. L., Orleans, C. S., George, L. K., & Brodie, H. K. H. (1979). *The importance of mental health services to general healthcare.* Cambridge, MA: Ballinger.

Kaplan, H. I., & Sadock, B. J. (Eds.). (1985). *Comprehensive textbook of psychiatry/IV.* Baltimore: Williams & Wilkins.

Manderscheid, R. W., & Sonnenschein, M. A. (Eds.). (1991). *Mental health, United States: 1990* (NIMH Pub. No. ADM 90-708). Washington, DC: U.S. Government Printing Office.

McLellan, A. T., Arndt, I. O., Metzger, D. S., Woody, G. E., & O'Brien, C.

P. (1993). The effects of psychosocial services in substance abuse treatment. *JAMA, 269,* 1953–1959.

Morris, J. A. (1994). The history of managed care and its impact on psychodynamic treatment. *Journal of Psychoanalysis and Psychotherapy, 11,* 129–137.

Morris, J. A. (1995a). Alcohol and other drug dependency treatment: A proposal for integration with primary care. *Alcoholism Treatment Quarterly, 13,* 45–56.

Morris, J. A. (1995b). Quality standards in corporate dominated health care. *The Independent Practitioner, 15,* 116–119.

Muszynski, I. L., Brady, J., & Sharfstein, S. S. (1987). *Economic fact book for psychiatry* (2nd ed.). Washington, DC: American Psychiatric Press.

Narrow, W. E., Regier, D. A., Rae, D. S., et al. (1993). Use of services by persons with mental and addictive disorders. *Archives of General Psychiatry, 50,* 95–107.

National Institute of Mental Health, Division of Biometry and Epidemiology. (1978). *Relation of occupancy rate to bed size and urban status—general hospital psychiatric inpatient units, 35.* Rockville, MD: National Institute of Mental Health.

National Mental Health Association. (1988). *Report of the National Action Commission on the mental health of rural Americans.* Alexandria, VA: Author.

National Rural Health Association. (1993). *Mental health and rural Americans: 1980–1993* (NIH Pub. No. 94-3500). Rockville, MD: National Institute of Mental Health, National Institutes of Health.

Nielsen, A. C., & Williams, T. A. (1980). Depression in ambulatory medical patients. *Archives of General Psychiatry, 37,* 999–1004.

Parlour, P. R., Young, L. M., Jones, L. R., & Brady, T. J. (1985). Mental health treatment and medical care utilization in a fee-for-service system: Outpatient mental health treatment following the onset of a chronic disease. *American Journal of Public Health, 73,* 422–429.

Paul, G. L., & Lentz, R. J. (1977). *Psychosocial treatments of chronic mental patients.* Cambridge, MA: Harvard University Press.

Redick, R. W. (1976). *Admission rates to federally funded community mental health centers, United States 1973* (Mental Health Statistical Note No. 126). Rockville, MD: National Institute of Mental Health.

Regier, D. A., Farmer, M. E., Rae, D. S., Locke, B. Z., Keith, S. J., Judd, L. L., & Goodwin, F. K. (1990). Comorbidity of mental disorders with alcohol and other drug abuse results from the Epidemiologic Catchment Area (ECA) study. JAMA, *264,* 2511–2518.

Regier, D. A., Goldberg, I. D., & Taube, C. A. (1978). The de facto U.S. mental health services system: A public perspective. *Archives of General Psychiatry, 35,* 685–693.

Regier, D. A., Myers, J. K., Kramer, M., Robins, L. N., Blazer, D. G., Hough, R. L., Eaton, W. W., & Locke, B. Z. (1984). The NIMH Epidemiologic Catchment Area program: Historical context, major objectives, and study population characteristics. *Archives of General Psychiatry, 41,* 934–941.

Robins, L. N., & Regier, D. A. (1990). *Psychiatric disorders in America.* New York: Free Press.

Rosenberg, J. (1986). *Policy forum: The personal stress problems of farmers and rural Americans (Summary report).* Forum sponsored by the National Institute of Mental Health and the Center for Agricultural and Rural Development of the Council of State Government.

Schulberg, H. C., Saul, M., McClelland, M., et al. (1985, December). Assessing depression in primary medical and psychiatric practices. *Archives of General Psychiatry, 42,* 1164–1170.

Schulberg, H. C., & Scott, C. P. (1991). Depression in primary care: Treating depression with interpersonal psychotherapy. In C. S. Austad & W. H. Berman (Eds.), *Psychotherapy in managed health care: The optimal use of time and resources* (pp. 153–170). Washington, DC: American Psychological Association.

Schuster, J. M. (1995). Psychiatric consultation in the general hospital emergency department. *Psychiatric Services, 46,* 555–557.

Shahinpour, N., Hollinger-Smith, L., & Perlia, M. A. (1995). The medical–psychiatric consultation liaison nurse. Meeting psychosocial needs of medical patients in the acute care setting. *Nursing Clinics of North America, 30,* 77–86.

Smith, G. R. (1993). Managed care, managed competition, and mental health. *Focus On Mental Health Services Research, 6,* 1.

Wallace, C. J., & Liberman, R. P. (1985). Social skills training for patients with schizophrenia: A controlled clinical trial. *Psychiatry Research, 15,* 239–247.

White, C. L., Bateman, A., Fisher, W. H., & Geller, J. L. (1995). Factors associated with admission to public and private hospitals from a psychiatric emergency screening site. *Psychiatric Services, 46,* 467–472.

Yank, G. R., Barber, J. W., Vieweg, W. V. R., Hundley, P. H., Spradlin, W. W., Harding, L. F., & Sutker, L. H. (1991). Virginia's experience with state–university collaboration. *Hospital and Community Psychiatry, 42,* 39–44.

III

Special Populations in Hospital Practice

Clinical Neuropsychology in the Rural Hospital

Paul L. Craig

Tersely defined, *neuropsychology* is the scientific study of the relation between brain function and behavior (Kolb & Whishaw, 1990). Clinical neuropsychology is the application of this body of knowledge to patients with known or suspected disorders of the central nervous system. This chapter describes the work of the clinical neuropsychologist, emphasizing the challenges of practicing in a rural setting.

History

Clinical neuropsychology was composed of a relatively small and tightly knit group of scientists–practitioners typically housed in medical school settings during the 1950s through the 1970s. The publication of Halstead's (1947) seminal book *Brain and Intelligence* represented an early hallmark in the development of this specialized field of scientific inquiry. Reitan and Davidson's (1974) edited text *Clinical Neuropsychology: Current Status and Applications*, assisted in catapulting neuropsychology from the arena of scientific inquiry into a field of clinical practice. Finally, Lezak's (1976) publication of the first edition of *Neuropsychological Assessment* provided a firm foundation for the development of clinical neuropsychology as a psychological specialty. During the late 1970s and early 1980s, a logarithmic increase in books, scientific journals, and professional associations concerned with neuropsychology occurred. For several years, the Division of Clinical Neuropsychology was one of the fastest-growing divisions in the American Psychological Association (APA). Likewise, the International Neuropsychological Association and the National Academy of Neuropsychology enjoyed dramatic increases in membership during the 1980s. Doctoral and postdoctoral training programs preparing specialists in the field of clinical neuropsychology have also enjoyed a similar rate of growth during recent years (Cripe, 1995). In 1981, the American Board of Clinical Neuropsychology was incorporated. This board developed into one of the nine specialty areas of practice subsumed under the American Board of Professional Psychology (ABPP). The ABPP diplomate has been recognized as a standard of excellence in psychology since its inception in 1947. Despite the meteoric rise of clinical neuropsychology as a field of specialty practice, virtually nothing has been written about the delivery of neuropsychological services in rural communities.

Neuropsychological Services

Patients seen for evaluation or treatment by a clinical neuropsychologist include those suffering from acquired disorders of the central nervous system (e.g., traumatic brain injury; Levin, Benton, & Grossman, 1982) as well as those suffering from developmental disorders interfering with normal brain functions (Spreen, Tupper, Risser, Tuokko, & Edgell, 1984). Neuropsychologists provide services in both the inpatient and outpatient arenas. Those benefiting from neuropsychological services include pediatric, adult, and gerontological patients. Clinical services rendered by neuropsychologists include assessment, consultation and education, and treatment.

Assessment

Within both inpatient and outpatient settings, neuropsychologists are commonly called on by physicians and other referral sources to evaluate neurocognitive abilities in patients suffering from known or suspected disorders of the brain. The neuropsychological evaluation typically includes a thorough clinical interview with the patient, family member, or other informants, as well as the administration of a series of neuropsychological tests that have been demonstrated to be sensitive to brain–behavior relationships. Although there is significant debate among neuropsychologists regarding the optimal battery of tests necessary to derive answers to specific referral questions, there is consensus that tests used in the clinical setting must demonstrate reliability and validity to discern patterns of cognitive impairment associated with disorders of brain functions (Franzen, 1989).

When evaluating acute inpatients, an abbreviated neuropsychological screening evaluation can sometimes be completed at bedside within an hour. With high-functioning patients who are suspected of having more subtle neurocognitive deficits, a complete neuropsychological evaluation can involve four to eight hours of testing using an extensive battery of standardized neuropsychological instruments.

Neurocognitive skills assessed in the neuropsychological evaluation include basic sensory and motor abilities, perceptual-motor skills, language functions, memory, higher level problem-solving and executive functions, as well as personality, emotional status, and motivational factors that may be influencing performance. The findings from the neuropsychological assessment are integrated into a consultation report. This report includes an overview of the patient's history, behavioral observations, interpretation of test performances, diagnostic impression, functional implications of the neurocognitive findings, and specific recommendations to benefit the patient in the context of maximizing adaptive functioning at home, in the classroom, on the job, or in the community. The neuropsychological assessment represents a snapshot of the patient's neurocognitive strengths and weaknesses at the time of evaluation. In the case of recently acquired disorders of the central nervous system, it is common to expect significant changes in neurocognitive abilities over time, necessitating serial reevaluations as the patient progresses in recovery (Levin, Grafman, & Eisenberg, 1987) or regresses in the context of a degenerative disorder, such as Alzheimer's disease (Adams, Craig, & Parsons, 1986).

Consultation and Education

In the hospital setting, neuropsychologists are frequently called on to consult with physicians, other health care providers, family members of patients, and other concerned individuals regarding the neurobehavioral implications of medical disorders involving the central nervous system. As a specialist among behavioral health providers, the neuropsychologist is uniquely trained and qualified to help patients and family members understand the current neurocognitive functional status demonstrated by a patient, and the range of outcomes predicated on a knowledge of the scientific research regarding neuropsychological changes over time among specific patients populations (e.g., Dikmen, Machamer, Temkin, & McLean, 1990). Likewise, the neuropsychologist can be of assistance with regard to community education and prevention efforts relative to preventable disorders of the brain. Dentists have engaged in a superlative effort at teaching the public good dental hygiene behaviors. Likewise, it is incumbent on neuropsychologists to participate in community education regarding importance of helmets, seatbelts, and avoidance of teratogenic substances such as alcohol during pregnancy. As a consultant and educator representing the rural hospital, the neuropsychologist assumes a relatively high profile as a specialized health service provider in the community.

Frequently, rural communities are unable to attract a full

complement of specialty physicians such as neurologists and physical medicine and rehabilitation physicians. In the context of serving the needs of the rural community, inclusion of a neuropsychologist on a rural hospital health care staff can fill an important niche relative to diagnosis and rehabilitation of brain-impaired patients.

Treatment

The neuropsychologist typically works in concert with a multidisciplinary team of rehabilitation specialists. The neuropsychologist is trained to provide cognitive rehabilitation services to assist patients with respect to recovery of brain functions following an insult to the central nervous system (Sohlberg & Mateer, 1989). To the extent that specific neurocognitive abilities cannot be restored, the neuropsychologist assists the patient in developing compensatory strategies to improve functioning despite the persisting deficits. For example, a traumatic brain injury patient with persisting memory deficits can be trained to systematically use a memory notebook to record important information rather than relying on impaired memory processes. Environmental changes are also frequently recommended by the neuropsychologist. Labels on cupboard doors can be quite helpful to the patient suffering from spatial memory deficits. There has been a significant amount of scientific debate regarding the efficacy of various forms of cognitive rehabilitation. In consideration of cost-effectiveness, it is incumbent on the neuropsychologists to provide these services in a pragmatic and individually relevant manner. For example, when providing cognitive rehabilitation services to a young adult leading a subsistence lifestyle in the Alaska Bush, it is important to recognize the irrelevance of many laboratory-oriented cognitive rehabilitation activities. Rather, the focus of cognitive rehabilitation with this type of patient may involve how to recall all of the steps necessary for safe operation of a chain saw or snow machine.

The neuropsychologist also brings an array of behavioral management strategies to the clinical setting (Meier, Benton,

& Diller, 1987). These skills are notably helpful in the inpatient environment. For example, when patients are emerging from coma and are agitated and confused during posttraumatic amnesia, behavioral management strategies associated with minimal stimulation protocols can be of great assistance in minimizing the use of neuroleptics or physical restraints for patient management. As might be expected, family members of agitated and confused patients are most thankful when their loved one is managed compassionately using state of the art minimal stimulation protocols rather than tied to a bed or increasingly obtunded secondary to major neuroleptics. In the rural community, good relations with individual families quickly translates into good community relations. As the patient progresses out of the confused and agitated state, the neuropsychologist's behavioral management skills can be of assistance with respect to motivating the brain-impaired patient to participate in treatment regimens and other therapy protocols, such as physical therapy or occupational therapy.

Psychotherapy is a useful form of treatment provided by the neuropsychologist. Although neuropsychological patients suffer from brain disorders, these patients can experience the full range of human emotions. Frequently, the psychosocial deficits caused by a neurocognitive disorder create significant levels of anxiety and sometimes paranoia in impaired patients as they attempt to navigate within their social environment. Brain-impaired patients can benefit from the psychotherapeutic alliance with the neuropsychologist as they attempt to develop a realistic understanding of their neurocognitive deficits, prognosis, and functional implications.

Family members and other concerned parties involved with a brain-impaired patient frequently require some psychotherapeutic intervention to assist them in coping with their grief as they attempt to accept the changes demonstrated by the patient. Given the knowledge regarding brain disorders and the advanced training in psychotherapy received by the clinical neuropsychologist, this professional is optimally prepared to respond to the rural family's needs as they learn about and attempt to cope with the consequences of an acquired brain disorder.

Professional Training and Credentialing

APA's Division of Clinical Neuropsychology established the Task Force on Education, Training, and Credentialing. In 1989, the task force promulgated a *Definition of Clinical Neuropsychologist* specifying that neuropsychology is a specialty field of practice at the doctoral level. A 1-year predoctoral internship is typically completed, as well as postdoctoral training and clinical experience specializing in neuropsychology. To comply with the definition promulgated by APA's Division of Clinical Neuropsychology, the independent practitioner of neuropsychology must have completed 2 or more years of appropriate supervised training applying neuropsychological services in a clinical setting.

An increasing number of clinical neuropsychologists are pursuing board certification through the American Board of Clinical Neuropsychology, the specialty board under the ABPP. Historically, only a minority of practicing clinical psychologists have sought board certification. For example, only 237 diplomates have been granted by the American Board of Clinical Neuropsychology (Directory of Diplomates, 1995).

However, an increasing number of practitioners are recognizing the importance of this credential and are choosing to participate in the peer evaluation process to achieve Diplomate status. The absence of board certification does not connote incompetence. Only a small minority of practicing neuropsychologists have pursued the credential. However, practitioners who have been granted the Diplomate from the American Board of Clinical Neuropsychology have been subjected to rigorous examination of credentials and clinical competence by leaders in the field.

The clinical neuropsychologist is steeped in the tradition of clinical psychology, including knowledge and training regarding theories of behavior, emotion, personality, and psychopathology. In addition, the clinical neuropsychologist receives specialty training involving neuroanatomy, neurophysiology, neuropathology, and brain–behavior relationships.

It is incumbent on the clinical neuropsychologist to stay abreast of the rapidly burgeoning scientific literature regarding brain–behavior relationships among specific patient populations. Although remaining abreast of this increasing body of knowledge has traditionally been difficult for the practitioner in rural settings, the advent of the personal computer and advances in telecommunications have dramatically improved the practitioner's access to current scientific findings pertinent to the practice of neuropsychology.

Similar to recruitment of specialist physicians, the rural community hospital may experience difficulty recruiting and retaining properly trained clinical neuropsychologists. However, there is an ever increasing number of young professionals completing their postdoctoral training in neuropsychology. Among these professionals, more and more are recognizing the merits of living and working in a rural community.

Use of Nondoctoral Personnel

Although some neuropsychologists prefer to personally administer the entire battery of neuropsychological tests in order to benefit from qualitative aspects of performance, it is an accepted and standard practice within the field to use nondoctoral technicians for routine administration of standardized neuropsychological tests ("Guidelines," 1989; "Statement," 1992). The neuropsychologist is responsible for the clinical interview with the patient, as well as selection and interpretation of the tests administered to the patient. However, a nondoctoral technician working under the direct supervision of the neuropsychologist can perform a variety of the routine testing procedures on behalf of the neuropsychologist to improve the cost-effectiveness of the evaluation service. Use of neuropsychometrists is a cost-effective strategy to extend the coverage of the neuropsychologist in the rural hospital setting.

Relationship With Other Health Service Providers

Within the hospital as well as in the outpatient setting, neuropsychologists are frequently called on by neurologists and other physicians to evaluate higher cortical processes of patients with known or suspected brain disorders. Neurologists are well prepared to engage in differential medical diagnosis among patients with suspected brain disorders, utilizing a broad array of laboratory and associated diagnostic procedures. The clinical neuropsychologist has specialized training and assessment techniques for purposes of delineating the extent to which a patient suffers from disruption in higher cortical functions secondary to a specific neurological disease process. In some instances, the neuropsychological evaluation is the most critical piece of clinical data used for differential diagnosis. For example, differential diagnosis of dementia of the Alzheimer's type among the elderly is commonly dependent on the findings gleaned in the context of the neuropsychological evaluation as requested by a neurologist (e.g., Fuld, 1984).

As suggested previously, the neuropsychologist typically participates in a multidisciplinary team of health service providers when practicing in the urban hospital. In addition to neurologists, members of the team can include a physical medicine and rehabilitation physician (i.e., physiatrist), speech and language pathologist, occupational therapist, physical therapist, rehabilitation nurse, social worker, recreational therapist, clergy, and of course the patient and his or her family. Ideally, all health service providers on the multidisciplinary team are capable of functioning collaboratively while tolerating the inevitable overlap of roles and skills. The successful rehabilitation team is able to focus on the goal of maximizing the functioning of the patient in the social environment. Of course, in the rural hospital setting, the full complement of rehabilitation specialists may not be available. Given the extensive training and experience received by the properly trained clinical neuropsychologist, inclusion of this specialist on the rehabilitation team in the rural hospital can help assure that all patients in need of rehabilitation services are handled competently and professionally.

Case Example: Clinical Involvement With a Patient

The following represents a typical scenario in which the clinical neuropsychologist would be an active participant in consultation and treatment in the hospital setting. A 22-year-old single man is admitted to the hospital emergency room following involvement in a multivehicle accident. The patient is acutely treated neurosurgically for a depressed temporal bone skull fracture and associated epidural hematoma. The neurosurgeon describes the patient as having a Glasgow Coma Score (Jennett & Bond, 1975) of 6 on admission to the emergency room. After the patient has been neurosurgically stabilized and is being treated in the Intensive Care Unit, the neurosurgeon writes an order requesting consultation from the neuropsychologist.

The neuropsychologist reviews the medical chart, performs a cursory bedside evaluation of the patient to assess responsiveness to the environment, and then contacts family members to obtain a more thorough psychosocial history. Likewise, the neuropsychologist uses this opportunity to begin educating the family regarding the nature and consequences of the patient's injury. The range of prognostic outcomes, including time frames and relative probability of occurrence, is discussed with the family. As the patient emerges from coma and becomes agitated, the neuropsychologist administers the Galveston Orientation and Amnesia Test (Levin, O'Donnell, & Grossman, 1979) on a regular basis to objectively determine when the patient is emerging from posttraumatic amnesia. Concurrently, the neuropsychologist institutes a minimal stimulation protocol to environmentally reduce agitation and hopefully minimize the need for use of physical restraints and psychopharmacological interventions.

After the patient has emerged from posttraumatic amnesia,

an initial neuropsychological assessment is performed. The neuropsychologist communicates these findings in the form of a written consult to the primary treating physician, as well as other rehabilitation health service providers working with the patient. These results are also communicated to the family and the patient in terms understandable to the lay person. Of course, disclosure of results is guided by and consistent with ethical and legal considerations regarding confidentiality. As the patient moves toward discharge from the inpatient setting, the neuropsychologist assists with smooth transition to outpatient therapies and helps the patient access appropriate rural community resources such as the vocational rehabilitation program servicing the community.

Neuropsychological reevaluation is completed after the patient has enjoyed several months of recovery. While progressing in recovery, the patient is encouraged to participate in outpatient therapeutic modalities, including psychotherapy services. Depending on the demographic characteristics of the patients, various community resources can be called on by the clinical neuropsychologist, including disability adjudicators at Social Security, special education personnel through the school district, pre-injury employers, independent living specialists, or other resources available within the rural community.

Recruitment

A few years ago, a hospital was attempting to recruit a neuropsychologist through a display advertisement in the employment section of the APA *Monitor*. The advertisement included a picture of a white rhinoceros with a caption suggesting that neuropsychologists are as rare as the elusive white rhino. This shortage of specialized personnel in clinical neuropsychology has improved during recent years as a consequence of the increasing number of training programs available (Cripe, 1995) and its increasing popularity as a specialty field of practice.

Classified advertisements in the APA *Monitor* can be an

effective strategy to communicate with the pool of neuro-psychologists seeking practice opportunities. Under ideal circumstances, having a board-certified clinical neuropsychologist on the staff of the rural hospital is most desirable. However, there are many properly trained and well qualified clinical neuropsychologists who have not chosen to seek board certification. It can be most challenging for a rural hospital administrator to discern the appropriateness of training, experience, and credentials of the professional purporting to provide neuropsychological services. In this context, it may be helpful to contact a local board-certified neuropsychologist to assist with review of credentials and competence in the context of the definition of a clinical neuropsychologist as promulgated by the APA Division of Clinical Neuropsychology ("Definition of a Clinical Neuropsychologist," 1989).

Conclusion

Clinical neuropsychology is a relatively young but rapidly growing field of specialization within the spectrum of health service providers. Inclusion of clinical neuropsychology services in the menu of specialty services available to patients at a rural community hospital can improve the quality of care provided to brain-impaired patients. Inclusion of the clinical neuropsychologist on the health service staff of an inpatient health care facility benefits the institution, the patients, and the perception of the institution within the larger community. By working collaboratively with other members of the multidisciplinary health care team, the neuropsychologist brings an important understanding of brain–behavior relationships to the evaluation and treatment of patients with known or suspected brain disorders.

References

Adams, R. L., Craig, P. L., & Parsons, O. A. (1986). Neuropsychology of dementia. *Neurologic Clinics, 4,* 387–404.

Cripe, L. L. (1995). Listing of training programs in clinical neuropsychology—1995. *The Clinical Neuropsychologist, 9,* 327–398.

Definition of *clinical neuropsychologist.* (1989). *The Clinical Neuropsychologist, 3,* 22.

Dikmen, S., Machamer, J., Temkin, N., & McLean, A. (1990). Neuropsychological recovery in patients with moderate to severe head injury: Two-year follow-up. *Journal of Clinical and Experimental Neuropsychology, 12,* 507–519.

Directory of Diplomates. (1995). Columbia, MO: American Board of Professional Psychology.

Franzen, M. D. (1989). *Reliability and validity in neuropsychological assessment.* New York: Plenum Press.

Fuld, P. A. (1984). Test profile of cholinergic dysfunction and of Alzheimer-type dementia. *Journal of Clinical Neuropsychiatry, 6,* 380–392.

Guidelines regarding the use of nondoctoral personnel in clinical neuropsychological assessment. (1989). *The Clinical Neuropsychologist, 3,* 23–24.

Halstead, W. C. (1947). *Brain and intelligence.* Chicago: University of Chicago Press.

Jennett, B., & Bond, M. (1975). Assessment of outcome after severe brain damage. A practical scale. *The Lancet, 1,* 480–484.

Kolb, B., & Whishaw, I. Q. (1990). *Fundamentals of human neuropsychology* (3rd ed.). New York: W. H. Freeman.

Levin, H. S., Benton, A. L., & Grossman, R. G. (1982). *Neurobehavioral consequences of closed head injury.* New York: Oxford University Press.

Levin, H. S., Grafman, J., & Eisenberg, H. M. (1987). *Neurobehavioral recovery from head injury.* New York: Oxford University Press.

Levin, H. S., O'Donnell, V. M., & Grossman, R. G. (1979). The Galveston Orientation and Amnesia Test: A practical scale to assess cognition after head injury. *Journal of Nervous and Mental Disease, 167,* 675–684.

Lezak, M. D. (1976). *Neuropsychological assessment.* New York: Oxford University Press.

Meier, M. J., Benton, A. L., & Diller, L. (1987). *Neuropsychological rehabilitation.* New York: Guilford Press.

Reitan, R. M., & Davidson, L. A. (1974). *Clinical neuropsychology: Current status and applications.* New York: Winston & Wiley.

Sohlberg, M. M., & Mateer, C. A. (1989). *Introduction to cognitive rehabilitation: Theory and practice.* New York: Guilford Press.

Spreen, O., Tupper, D., Risser, A., Tuokko, H., & Edgell, D. (1984). *Human developmental neuropsychology.* New York: Oxford University Press.

Statement regarding the use of nondoctoral personnel for neuropsychological assessment. (1992). *The Clinical Neuropsychologist, 6,* 256.

The Wellness of Women: Implications for the Rural Health Care Provider

Sue A. Kuba and Mary Beth Kenkel

Women's health concerns are becoming increasingly more important to hospitals and health care providers for several reasons. Surveys indicate that women make most health care decisions for all members of their families. They decide which pediatrician, hospital, and health care plan to use. They make the appointments and often transport their children and parents to health care services. Often they are the family researchers of health information and self-help health care. Women have therefore become a central focus for measures of consumer satisfaction with the health care industry (Collins, 1994; Helgeson, 1994; Travis, 1988).

In addition, a woman is more likely than a man to seek medical and other health services for her own personal needs (Travis, 1988). Some authors speculate that this is created by a woman's greater willingness to admit physical weakness when compared with men (Helgeson, 1994). Others suggest that women seek medical help for psychological difficulties such as depression or anxiety (van Dulmen, Fennis, Mokkink, van der Velden, & Bleijenberg, 1994). This may be especially true for women in rural areas where use of mental health services still carries much stigma.

Another reason women access care more is a result of some conditions being more common in women than men. Conditions such as rheumatoid arthritis, chronic fatigue syndrome, multiple sclerosis, and lupus each present a difficult diagnostic and treatment picture (Hotopf & Wessely, 1994; Neely & Borden, 1994; Smith & Wallston, 1992). These conditions necessitate frequent visits to the primary care physician and may involve extensive diagnostic procedures prior to the start of treatment. Women's reproductive health concerns also require frequent physician contact and account for a substantial portion of hospital days (Abbey, Andrews, & Halman, 1991; Bloom, 1994).

For all of these reasons, hospital administrators and health care marketers have increasingly targeted women's health. The response has been positive. Women respond well to services that are designed for their specific needs (Silverman, 1988). This is especially true in the boundary where medical and psychological health care interact. Women are more likely to speak openly about their concerns when they feel their unique perspective is understood. This perspective includes attention to the psychosocial effects of physical illness as well to obtaining accurate information about the physical illness itself (Genero, Jordon, Goldstein, Elliot, & McMurray, 1994; Shapiro, Boggs, Melamed, & Graham-Pole, 1992). As women have gained greater confidence in themselves, they have become more demanding consumers. A woman's decision to use a particular health care institution for herself and her family will depend on her perception of that institution as holistic and psychosocially responsive.

In this chapter, we discuss the unique issues raised by women's health care in a rural environment, including (a) inclusion of a woman's perspective in health care delivery, (b) community health care education for rural women, (c) women's support groups, and (d) a biopsychosocial approach to women's health. Such information should provide you with practical approaches that will increase sensitivity to women's health in your community and demonstrate the role of psychologists in such interventions.

The Importance of Including Women's Health Care Perspective

The purchasers and consumers of health care make choices based on three criteria: the cost of care, satisfaction with care, and the quality of care. The inclusion of the women's perspective outlined above—one that expects accurate information from health care providers and attention to psychosocial elements of health conditions ensures fulfillment of all of these criteria.

First, it has been well established that various psychological and psychosocial interventions are effective in reducing medical costs. For example, surgery preparation procedures that include such components as providing relevant information to the surgery patient and teaching relaxation and other coping strategies have been associated with faster patient recovery, fewer postoperative medical complications, and reductions in pain-relieving medications and postoperative hospital days (Anderson, 1987; Devine & Cook, 1983; Mumford, Herbert, Glass, Patrick, & Curdon, 1984).

As health care plans reduce the allowable hospital days for a number of different procedures (e.g., obstetrics), rural hospitals will need to find cost-effective ways of reducing hospital stays while maintaining a high quality of care. Better preparation of patients and their families for hospital procedures, and outpatient follow-up care, will help in this effort to control costs. This will often require the use of a diverse team of health care professionals with a strong emphasis on the behavioral and psychosocial components of health care treatment.

As inpatient hospital days are reduced and census drops, hospitals increasingly will need to make available an array of medical treatment options for their patients. Less intensive and less costly care arrangements will need to be developed so that rural hospitals can continue to compete with the larger urban hospitals. Rural hospitals may become organizers of integrated health care systems, providing for all of patients' health care needs. This approach often proves more satisfying to patients, circumventing the need to visit several health care professionals who have little communication among themselves.

Such integrated care creates a more holistic approach to health, an approach women particularly value. In this integrated holistic approach, patients are able to obtain medical and psychosocial interventions for acute health problems, support for chronic conditions, and preventative health care.

Because their population base is small, rural hospitals cannot develop the specialized medical centers (e.g., diabetes center, cardiac center) popular in urban hospitals. However, they can create and utilize the same type of biopsychosocial approach that is used in these settings by developing collaborative multidisciplinary health care teams of professionals who subscribe to and implement that approach. The team (often consisting of a physician, nurse, physical therapist, nutritionist, psychologist, and social worker) find strategies for dealing with the physical, social, emotional, nutritional, and economic aspects of the health condition. For example, in the treatment of diabetes, the physician prescribes and monitors the patient's medical treatment; the nutritionist develops menu plans with the patient; the psychologist helps the patient develop strategies for adhering to the treatment and deals with the emotional and social effects of a changed diet and lifestyle; and the physical therapist develops and monitors a healthy and reasonable exercise program to control weight.

This same strategy can be applied to any number of other acute and chronic health conditions, heart attacks or heart disease, arthritis, and cancer treatment. The key is in creating a team that can apply its skills across a variety of medical problems. In addition, the members of the team must subscribe to a biopsychosocial model rather than view the health problems through the lens of their own discipline model (e.g., biological, psychological, or social) and be able to communicate across disciplines (McDaniel, 1995).

Such a multipronged approach to treatment also leads to a higher quality of care. For example, studies have found that the rate of nonadherence to medical regimens is quite high. For simple regimens (e.g., adhering to a prescribed treatment of oral medicine), 20% or more of patients will not follow treatment. That number can soar to 90% when the treatment is complex and involves greater lifestyle changes, such as exercise, dieting, and relaxation (Becker, 1990). It is more likely that treatment will be adhered to, and consequently be more efficacious, when obstacles (emotional, social, and behavioral) to treatment compliance have been addressed through a multifaceted treatment approach. Therefore, the inclusion of women's health care perspective in hospital care can positively and powerfully affect the cost of care, patient satisfaction, and the quality of care. In the following sections, we describe strategies for incorporating this holistic, multifaceted approach to women's health.

Community Health Education
for Rural Women

Rural hospitals can begin to create women's health services in cost-effective and highly visible ways. Generally, three different levels of service are recommended. These include free educational seminars, small time limited educational discussion groups, and self-help or support groups. The development of these services for specific rural areas can easily be designed by a community-oriented psychologist in consultation with hospital staff and health care providers. The initial step is the development of a community-based assessment to determine the overriding women's health concerns in the local area. Do the women in the area worry more about access to legal and safe abortion or in-home services for elderly parents? Are they high users of family planning services, concerned about chemical dependency, or more likely to have an eating disorder?

Surveys of the women in the community would be supplemented by interviews with primary health care providers, members of the clergy, and existing mental health providers. Such an assessment should provide epidemiological information about the primary health concerns of the women in the community. It should also give some indication of priority rankings and frequencies of those concerns. The next steps in developing women's health-based services would naturally flow from this needs assessment. The very act of completing such an assessment contributes to the perception of the health care institution as one that is concerned about women's health needs.

Selection of 5 to 10 topics from among those issues will provide the basis for initial free community health seminars, sponsored by the hospital. In these seminars, experts lecture on topics such as breast cancer prevention, caretaking and self-care, women's issues in HIV and AIDs, eating disorders and teenage girls, development and adherence to personal exercise programs, and so forth. Information about seminars can be formatted as a brochure with the hospital logo and wide community distribution. A local newspaper may have a calendar for listing such events. Marketing should occur through medical staff members' offices, schools, local service organizations, churches, beauty salons, and health clubs. Most organizations will gladly distribute information on such free seminars. To be successful such seminars need to occur locally and provide low fee child care. Seasonal topics may be especially successful (e.g., cold weather and depression). In rural communities, privacy becomes a primary concern. Opportunities for anonymous questions might be created through write-in questions placed in an inconspicuous place during the break. The presenter should allow for individual questions after the presentation.

Finally, an evaluation form requesting suggestions for future seminars should be provided. Many health and mental health care providers are willing to give such lectures in exchange for free publicity and an ongoing referral relationship with the hospital. A psychologist consultant may provide some of these lectures or select other providers to participate in this process. Feedback about specific presenters should be maintained and used to plan the women's health educational seminars for the next year or season.

Once there is a successful community education program

geared toward women's interests and needs, the intensity of these services may increase. Time-limited psychoeducational interventions are usually the next step. These are classes, facilitated by mental health and health care professionals, that address basic emotional and physical concerns about health care issues. The decision about which classes to offer will depend on the information gained from the first two steps, the community needs assessment and the educational seminars. Generally, it is best to begin with one or two classes with a high chance for success. An example is a class for new mothers and their infants. This class requires 6 to 10 weekly meetings and meets for about an 1.5 hours. The class focuses on the challenges and joys of new motherhood. It includes topics related to successful parenting skills, management of stress, how to deal with sleep deprivation, finding time for self, and so forth. Each week presents a different topic, some basic information and a discussion of individual needs and concerns. Such interventions have been shown to decrease depression in new mothers and provide contact among individuals at similar life stages (Rhodes, Contreras, & Mangelsdorf, 1994). It is important to have qualified staff members provide services where content may become emotional in nature. Again the issue of privacy is primary. Many women will attend such a class if the content is not too threatening and is presented as educational in nature. Fees may be charged for such classes. Customary amounts will vary for your area but should be in the neighborhood of $10 to $20 per week. This educational offering should be perceived as a not-for-profit service, which will promote outpatient and tertiary health services. Other potential topics for rural services include relationship enrichment for couples, menopause and its treatment, stress reduction for women, help for the chemically dependent, and healthy cooking and appetite management.

The third phase of community education intervention includes the development of support group services for those with ongoing physical–social–psychological needs. Usually these groups will be created to confront a common chronic physical illness, with psychological ramifications (Chung &

Magraw, 1992). They operate continuously due to the nature of the content. Fees usually vary from $20 to $35 per session. Sessions usually last for at least 1.5 hours. An example is a breast cancer support group.

In addition to concerns about mortality, the woman with breast cancer faces an assault on her sense of femininity and womanhood (Apfel, Love, & Kalinowski, 1994). Often family and friends are uncertain about how to respond to the threat of physical and emotional loss. Male partners or husbands are particularly uncertain about their role as a support to the woman. Her sexuality is often affected. A family support group that provides education and a place for information sharing among those close to the woman with breast cancer may also be helpful. The content of support groups is more emotionally laden, as the woman and her family are struggling with an ongoing and difficult health crisis. Extensive information has usually already been obtained. The educational function of the women's support group often involves resource sharing and specifics about response to their treatment (e.g., living through chemotherapy). Women will continue to attend such a group however if it becomes a place where their greatest fears and anxieties are addressed. Few friends or partners find it easy to discuss approaching death with a woman with metastasized cancer. Women have difficulty talking about feelings of disfigurement from mastectomy with even close female friends.

The support group creates a safe place for exploration of such feelings in a confidential environment. Such services need to be provided by a mental health professional whose ethical code calls for strict confidentiality. He or she must be a person who can create an understanding of the need for such confidentiality among group members, who can establish boundaries and rules for the group's functioning and confront those who violate such boundaries. Such groups should be ongoing, with a period for enrollment every 4 to 6 months. This gives the group time to develop trust and allows new members to enter with others who have not been a part of the group. Location and time of the group need to be dependent on convenience and privacy. Sometimes a women's group is best held during daytime hours.

The needs assessment should give some indication when women feel they are most willing to take time for their own emotional needs. Marketing these types of support groups will depend heavily on physician referral. The support group leader needs to be an individual who can network with physicians and provide useful information about the importance of such support. There are data available to demonstrate the positive impact of social support on the physical health of patients. Providing this research to physicians in a way that is sensitive to their own expertise may require the supervision of a community-oriented psychologist consultant. A successful individual will be invited to speak to the local medical association and ought to be a member of the medical staff, where information can be shared more informally. Marketing may also be targeted directly to the public through community service announcements or regular hospital publications. Each may be announced in the physicians' newsletters or a mailing to providers' offices. Sometimes, front office staff are the best referral sources for such groups. Receptionists who are aware of such offerings may pass this information to patients who are struggling with the emotional consequences of illness.

Many types of support groups have been successful. The community needs assessment will indicate the specific needs of the local area. Some important support groups to consider include those for caretakers (women responsible for someone with a chronic illness such as Alzheimer's disease), adolescents with eating disorders, chemical dependency in the family, older single women and widows, and women living with cancer or other chronic illnesses.

In developing a comprehensive educational outreach program such as the one described here, it is important to develop partnerships with other institutions in the community. Educational seminars and psychoeducational interventions may be offered in the multipurpose room of a church or school or at the local bank community service room. Y.W.C.A.s or other health facilities may welcome a partnership that provides easy access to health education for its female members. Often these sites provide child care, so that separate arrangements are not necessary. Creating such educational services for women in the rural community will provide a link to women who serve as the primary health care decision maker.

The Biopsychosocial Approach to Women's Health Care

In addition to providing psychoeducational programs and self-help and support groups, rural hospitals also can address the psychosocial aspects of women's health needs in both inpatient and outpatient services. This is the arena in which psychologists and other mental health professionals can contribute much to negotiating that interface between the physical and psychological aspects of health problems.

The occurrence, frequency, course, and severity of many physical ailments are influenced by psychosocial variables. For example, the occurrence and frequency of irritable bowel syndrome, rheumatoid arthritis, tension headaches, and cardiac arrest have been associated with psychological stress. Symptom severity and recurrences of such chronic conditions as chronic fatigue syndrome and multiple sclerosis also are more likely to occur under periods of high stress.

For these and other conditions, patients can benefit much from psychological interventions that provide patients with the ability to identify, reduce, and cope with stressors in their lives. A variety of psychological treatments have been helpful in this regard: short-term therapy, relaxation training, hypnosis, cognitive therapy, and biofeedback. In addition, some health problems that cause minor or major disruptions in patients' lives also respond well to psychophysiological interventions. For example, urinary incontinence is a major reason for the institutionalization of the elderly, many of whom are women. However, this condition responds well to a short course of biofeedback. This treatment may be especially helpful to the rural patient who may have limited options for nursing care facilities and may prefer staying in the family home.

Psychologists can also provide consultation to physicians for understanding and dealing with the emotional and interpersonal aspects of physical conditions. While all patients benefit from this attention, women especially expect and feel more satisfied with discussion of the psychosocial aspects of health problems. This need can occur in any hospital department, for example, in connection with breast surgery, low weight births, seriously ill children, Alzheimer's patients, and so forth. Especially in rural areas, the physician is looked to as the person to attend to all the patient's needs. This expectation can be extremely taxing and draining to the physician, often contributing to physician burnout and difficulties in retaining physicians in rural areas. Physicians may find great relief if they feel that the psychologist can assist them by attending to the emotional needs and concerns of the patient and the family, allowing physicians to devote most of their concentration to the biomedical treatment (McDaniel, 1995).

In addition to the impact of physical problems on psychosocial functioning, there are a number of psychological problems that have significant deleterious effects on physical health. For example, eating disorders, including anorexia and bulimia, are most prevalent among young women and teenage girls. The incidence of these conditions range from 1% to 3% among adolescent and young female adults (*Diagnostic and Statistical Manual of Mental Disorders,* 4th ed. [*DSM-IV*], APA, 1994).

Left untreated, eating disorders can result in extreme weight loss, dehydration, malnutrition, cardiac malfunctions, and even death. Early signs of eating disorders are often overlooked by physicians or are attributed to a "phase" in the teenager's life. In addition, patients with anorexia are often resistant to treatment, often believing, as a result of their distorted body image, that their emaciated bodies are still "too fat."

The best approach to treatment is through a multidisciplinary team consisting of a physician, psychologist, and nutritionist who can address both the medical and psychological needs of the individual. In severe cases, hospitalization is usually required to treat the medical complications and gain environmental control over the eating behavior. Intensive residential or outpatient treatment then follows.

Similar health-threatening effects can result from depression, one of the most prevalent psychological disorders among women. Women with depression usually seek out their physicians for treatment. However, physicians often fail to properly diagnose this condition, or, when they do correctly diagnose, give subtherapeutic dosages of antidepressants. Psychologists, and other mental health professionals, can assist in making a proper diagnosis and recommending a course of treatment. Psychotherapy has been found to be very effective with unipolar depression; major depression and bipolar depressions usually require psychotropic medications in addition to psychotherapy.

To avoid costly diagnostic procedures and ineffective courses of treatment, proper and efficient diagnosis is also necessary in a number of other conditions common to women that have substantial physical and psychological symptoms: chronic fatigue syndrome; anxiety disorders, with and without panic attacks; somatizing disorder; and substance abuse. Because of their extensive training in assessment and psychiatric diagnosis, psychologists can provide consultation in these difficult diagnostic cases. Early, accurate diagnosis can prevent the application of ineffective courses of treatment and frustration on the part of the patient and health care provider.

Conclusion

There are many effective ways for using a biopsychosocial model in treating women's health care problems. Such a model will not only provide a higher quality of care but also will respond to women's interests in a more holistic approach to health. By using this approach, the rural hospital will implement the integrated care model which is finding wide support. Other health care services (e.g., rehabilitation, vision care, and dental care) can easily be assimilated into this approach to provide rural residents with total and coordinated health care in their local communities.

References

Abbey, A., Andrews, F. M., & Halman, L. J. (1991). Gender's role in response to infertility. *Psychology of Women Quarterly, 15,* 295–316.

American Psychiatric Association. (1994). *Diagnostic and Statistical Manual of Mental Disorders* (4th ed.). Washington, DC: Author.

Anderson, E. A. (1987). Preoperative preparation for cardiac surgery facilitates recovery, reduces psychological distress, and reduces the incidence of acute postoperative hypertension. *Journal of Consulting and Clinical Psychology, 55,* 513–520.

Apfel, R. J., Love, S. M., & Kalinowski, B. H. (1994). Keep abreast: Women and breast cancer in context. In M. P. Mirkin (Ed.), *Women in context: Toward a feminist reconstruction of psychotherapy* (pp. 217–236). New York: Guilford.

Becker, M. H. (1990). Theoretical models of adherence and strategies for improving adherence. In S. A. Shumaker, E. B. Schron, J. K. Ockene, C. T. Parker, J. L. Probstfield, and J. M. Wolle (Eds.), *Handbook of health behavior change* (pp. 5–43). New York: Springer.

Bloom, J. B. (1994). The counter revolution: Sex, politics, and the new reproductive technologies. In M. P. Mirkin (Ed.), *Women in context: Toward a feminist reconstruction of psychotherapy* (pp. 284–309). New York: Guilford Press.

Chung, J. Y., & Magraw, M. M. (1992). A group approach to psychosocial issues faced by HIV positive women. *Hospital and Community Psychiatry, 43,* 891–894.

Collins, K. S. (1994, May). *The Commonwealth Fund Survey of women's health.* Paper presented at the American Psychological Association conference on "Psychosocial and Behavioral Factors in Women's Health: Creating an Agenda for the 21st Century," Washington, DC.

Devine, E. C., & Cook, T. D. (1993). A meta-analysis of effects of psychoeducational interventions on length of postsurgical hospital stay. *Nursing Research, 32,* 267–274.

Genero, N. P., Jordon, J., Goldstein, L. H., Elliot, D., & McMurray, J. E. (1994, May). *Promoting well-being through relationships in community, inpatient, and educational contexts.* Paper presented at the American Psychological Association Conference on "Psychosocial and Behavioral Factors in Women's Health: Creating an Agenda for the 21st Century," Washington, DC.

Helgeson, V. S. (1994). Relation of agency and communion to well-being: Evidence and potential explanations. *Psychological Bulletin, 116,* 412–428.

Hotopf, M., & Wessely, S. (1994). Viruses, neurosis and fatigue. *Journal of Psychosomatic Research, 38,* 499–514.

McDaniel, S. (1995). Collaboration between psychologists and family physicians: Implementing the biopsychosocial model. *Professional Psychology: Research and Practice, 26,* 117–122.

Mumford, E., Herbert, J., Glass, G. V., Patrick, C., & Curdon, T. (1984). A new look at evidence about reduced cost of medical utilization following mental health treatment. *American Journal of Psychiatry, 141,* 1145–1158.

Neely, F. W., & Borden, K. A. (1994, May). *Autoimmune disease: Issue for research and treatment.* Paper presented at the American Psychological Association's conference on "Psychosocial and Behavioral Factors in Women's Health: Creating an Agenda for the 21st Century," Washington, DC.

Rhodes, J. E., Contreras, J. M., & Mangelsdorf, S. C. (1994). Natural mentor relationships among latino adolescent mothers: Psychological adjustment, moderating processes, and the role of early parental acceptance. *American Journal of Community Psychology, 22,* 211–227.

Shapiro, D. E., Boggs, S. R., Melamed, B. G., & Graham-Pole, J. (1992). The effect of varied physician affect on recall, anxiety, and perceptions in women at risk for breast cancer: An analogue study. *Health Psychology, 11,* 61–66.

Silverman, P. R. (1988). Widow to widow: A mutual help program for the widowed. In Price et al. (Eds.), *Fourteen ounces of prevention* (pp. 175–186). Washington, DC: American Psychological Association.

Smith, C. A., & Wallston, K. A. (1992). Adaptation in patients with chronic rheumatoid arthritis: Application of a general model. *Health Psychology, 11,* 151–162.

Travis, C. B. (1988). *Women and health psychology: Biomedical issues.* Hillsdale, NJ: Erlbaum.

van Dulmen, A. M., Fennis, J. F. M., Mokkink, H. G. A., van der Velden, H. G. M., & Bleijenberg, G. (1994). Doctors' perceptions of patients' cognitions and complaints in irritable bowel syndrome at an outpatient clinic. *Journal of Psychosomatic Research, 38,* 581–590.

Rural Hospital Addictions Screening and Treatment

Jerry A. Morris and James G. Hill

As noted in chapter 6 (The Rural Psychologist in the Hospital Emergency Room), 10 out of 100 people will suffer a mental disorder (Kaplan & Sadock, 1985; Regier et al., 1984), and another 20 will suffer from substance abuse or dependence (Reiger et al., 1984; Reiger et al., 1990). Over half of all United States citizens will require psychological intervention (Reiger et al., 1984). Many of these individuals will suffer serious and persistent mental illness and will be unable to work (Barker et al., 1989).

In addition, there are approximately 46 million smokers in the United States, and many of them are addicted. When they are added to the figures just discussed, the numbers are staggering. Of course, many who are addicted to nicotine are also addicted to other substances. Hoffman and Slade (1992) in an article titled "Addressing Tobacco in Chemical Dependency Treatment" explored the reasons for inclusion of nicotine when treating other addictions. They enumerated the following reasons for addressing the problem of nicotine dependence: (a) It is an important cause of preventable death in substance abuse patients; (b) failing to address nicotine addiction undermines the treatment of other addictions; (c) many patients want to work on nicotine in conjunction with other addictions; (d) embedding nicotine addiction treatment in other addiction treatment helps overcome the possibility of nonreimbursement for nicotine addiction; (e) tobacco smoke pollution (secondary smoking) causes lung cancer, heart disease, and other problems; (f) relapse to nicotine use and de novo nicotine dependence occur among patients admitted to treatment programs for other dependencies; (g) it is against the law for adolescents in treatment programs to be allowed (or encouraged) to smoke; and (h) smoking can be a cue for other drug use, and smoking has often been paired closely with alcohol and drug abuse. As the above points demonstrate, the treatment of addictions has complex programmatic and therapeutic implications. This chapter reviews the cost-effectiveness of hospital treatment programs, models of treatment programs, and case examples to illustrate the overall efficacy of integrating substance abuse programs within rural hospital settings.

Cost-Effectiveness of Psychological Interventions

The high prevalence of substance abuse and mental illness indicates that between 1 in 7 to 1 in 4 individuals entering a primary health care system will have a diagnosable substance abuse, mental health problem, or both (Morris & Wise, 1992). Data covering the employed population in the United States (age 18 and over) indicate that 10.3% of men and 4.1% of women are alcohol dependent (Parker & Harford, 1992). Furthermore, these authors noted that 3.9% of men and 1.0% of women are severely chemically dependent. Many others will have a physical illness that is maintained by their behavior or related to lifestyle.

It has been noted that the top risks to good health in the United States (smoking, diet, alcohol, unintentional injuries, suicide, violence, and unsafe sex) are behavioral problems. Some of these behavioral problems give rise to addictive patterns. Psychological and addictions interventions are more appropriate than medical services for these patients (VandenBos, 1993).

The total economic costs of alcohol abuse and dependence for 1990 were estimated to be $98.6 billion with medical care costs estimated at $10.5 billion. Psychological and addictive behaviors resulting in medical care, or failure to treat the behavioral aspects of medical care, add additional costs (Hartman-Stein & Reuter, 1993; Rice, 1993).

Many physical diseases are related to behavioral and lifestyle management, and to overall psychological health (Cummings & Follette, 1968; Follette & Cummings, 1967). Research in this area has given rise to the concept of "medical offset," demonstrated when nonmedical treatment interventions cause a resulting decrease in medical usage and costs. Even when medical interventions have proven effective, medical noncompliance has demonstrated reduction in positive treatment outcome (Janis, 1984; Krantz & Glass, 1984; Leventhal, Zimmerman, & Gutman, 1984). Parallel psychological intervention often improves medical compliance and ultimately increases both medical and psychological effects.

Targeting mental health interventions to Medicaid patients with substance abuse disorders reduced medical care costs as much as $514 per person (15%) per year over a 5-year period. Medical costs for Medicaid patients who had substance abuse disorders but who did not receive mental health treatment increased 91% over that same period (Cummings, Dorken, Pallak, & Henke, 1990). Counseling and mental health components are necessary to treat compulsive, addictive processes such as eating disorders; smoking; and reckless, thrill-seeking behaviors that negatively affect long-term physical health.

It is becoming clear that a coordinated team and case-management approach is most treatment and cost-effective (Baker, Jodrey, Intagliatia, & Straus, 1993; Durell, Lechtenberg, Corse, & Frances, 1993; McLellan, Arndt, Metzger, Woody, & O'Brien, 1993). In a primary care center or hospital setting, the doctor of medicine or doctor of psychology acting as a team leader, emergency room screener, or hospital department head will need to have the philosophical and technical flexibility to work in multi-disciplinary team treatment and referral networks. Doctors of medicine must be free to assign treatment interventions to doctors of psychology who act as the attending practitioner coordinating the services of substance abuse counselors and mental health, educational, and case-management specialists. The psychologist will need to be available on staff and daily rotations in the hospital, and committed to assuming the responsibility for the addicted individual's total care, thus releasing the physician from the responsibility and time-consuming process of coordinating the case. Clinical leaders of the future working in multidisciplinary teams will be able to effect the highest quality of care in the least costly configuration (Mazade, 1990).

Evidence is mounting that the more counseling and psychosocial services a patient in some treatment populations receives the better the outcome. This is particularly apparent in the treatment of substance abuse and related disorders (Baker et al., 1993; Durell et al., 1993; McLellan et al., 1993). Increasingly, primary care physicians, psychologists, psychiatrically trained nurses, substance abuse counselors, and clinical and administrative social workers are collaborating to deliver effective coordinated care on the front lines of health care (Boydston, 1983; Broskowski, 1980; Buie, 1990; Burns, Burke, & Ozarin, 1983; Candib & Glenn, 1983; Celenza & Fenton, 1981; Dym & Berman, 1986; Enright & Blue, 1989). To do so, doctors of medicine and psychology must gain an understanding of the strengths and limits of their respective education and training; scope of practice; and the enabling legislation, rules, and regulations that allow collaboration (APA Rural Health Task Force, 1994).

There is strong evidence that alcoholism, particularly in its early stages, is poorly recognized in general medical practice settings and in hospitals with only physician diagnosticians available (Bradley, 1992; Brown, Carter, & Gordon, 1987; Coulehan, Zettler-Segal, Block, McClelland, & Schulberg, 1987; Moore & Malitz, 1986; Reid, Webb, Hennrikus, Fahey, & Sanson-Fisher, 1986; Schuckit, 1987; Umbrecht-Schneiter, Santora, & Moore, 1991). Generally, the prevalence of alcoholism and alcohol abuse in hospitalized patients has ranged from 4% to 70%, with most studies reporting these problems in one of four admissions (Baird, Burge, & Grant, 1989; Graham, 1991;

Hiller, Mombour, & Mittlehammer, 1989; Jarman & Kellet, 1979; Moore, 1971). The recidivism costs and general economic and health consequences of this underdiagnosing and treating are tremendous (Chan, Pristach, & Welte, 1994).

A holistic, integrated approach to substance abuse, family mental health, and physical disorders will emerge as the treatment of choice, one that is compatible with organized health care delivery systems that are concerned with demonstrated outcome and cost-effectiveness. Effective intervention for addicted individuals will necessitate a new primary health care model with the rural hospital at the hub of the wheel.

To reduce costs by making arrangements with facilities that offer comprehensive services, managed-care purchasers prefer contacts with hospitals and health care facilities that are "one stop shops." This pressure will influence many rural hospitals competing for area control to add psychologists to enhance their capacity to diagnose, treat, refer, and case manage substance-abusing patients.

The hospital will be pushed by managed care to include a multidisciplinary staff offering comprehensive services: diagnosis, stabilization, mobilization of family and community resources, and transfer and placement tracking in comprehensive outpatient treatment systems. Patient primary care needs will require that the hospitals and clinics be staffed by physicians and nurses, psychologists, social workers, and substance abuse counselors. The psychologist—as the premier doctoral mental health professional who is capable of collaborating with the primary care physician, performing in a cost-efficient manner, and willing to settle in the rural community—is the logical choice for the role of attending doctor and team leader for patients entering the hospital system with addiction as the primary disorder. The National Academy of Sciences Committee for the Study of Treatment and Rehabilitation Services for Alcoholism and Alcohol Abuse noted, "The committee urges strongly that a financial mechanism be developed to fund brief therapy outside of, as well as within, the context of funding for medical or medically-supervised services" (Mazade, 1990, p. 235).

Emerging Models

In 1980 the average family (four members) in the United States paid $1,742 for health care, and by the year 2000 some estimates indicate that the annual per family bill will be $9,397 ("Health Care," 1993). In 1991, families in New York paid an annual average of $5,585. President Clinton's Health Security Plan to reduce such costs called for an estimated $3,600 to $4,500 per family for the first year with likely adjustments each consecutive year (White House Domestic Policy Council, 1993).

White House consultants Ira Magaziner and Hillary Clinton indicated that $150 to $200 billion, or 20% of the nation's health care budget, is wasted on excessive administrative costs and unnecessary medical testing (Sperry, 1993). The government considered a national managed-care system as the vehicle to attempt to solve the problem (Koyanagi, Manes, Surles, & Goldman, 1993). Health care interest groups are laboring to ensure that the system does not overemphasize strictly biological interventions while neglecting psychological interventions and management of behavioral patterns causing many biological problems. There are estimates from the National Center for Policy Analysis that the long-term care component of the White House Plan and subsequent spin-off designs would have added $21 billion to the budget. Experts maintained that this is a dramatic underestimation (Merline, 1993).

Regardless of the numbers one believes or cites, it is clear that the health care system will move toward measurable and comparable alternative models of service delivery, efficiency, and a more rational basis of planning and health policy analysis. In recent years there has been a shift of patient care to settings outside of hospitals (Eichmann, Griffin, Lyons, Larson, & Finkel, 1992). To continue to provide leadership, advanced diagnosis, and protection from disaster in the most serious and difficult cases, the rural community hospital must move toward further integration with available outpatient centers, multidisciplinary staffing and approaches, more comprehensive diagnosis and treatment of behavioral and substance abuse disorders, and shortened lengths of stay.

In the arena of behavioral health and substance abuse, the hospital will be pressed to complete medical, psychological, and substance abuse diagnosis and stabilization in increasingly compressed lengths of stay. Within 1 to 3 days of admission, the hospital will have to accomplish medical evaluation and detoxification, psychological and family assessment, neuropsychological assessment, reduction of denial and projection defenses, location of outpatient and aftercare resources, and the completion of placement arrangements.

Increasingly, the hospital's effectiveness in substance abuse cases will be measured by the attending practitioner's ability to move rapidly from diagnosing and stabilizing the patient to arranging outpatient or day treatment placement to maintain sobriety, care for comorbid mental illness, address family and community dysfunction, and minimize the risk of rehospitalization. Self-help and support group approaches will be useful but will not be comprehensive enough to accomplish these tasks (Morris, 1994).

Case History

The following case example will demonstrate how effective short-term hospitalization, and an effective collaboration between physician and psychologist, can aid patient care.

Eileen, a mood-disordered recovering alcoholic, was given a minor tranquilizer by her psychiatrist. The psychiatrist had not reviewed the patient's social history or psychological evaluation. The tranquilizer resulted in a secondary addiction and Eileen developed panic attacks related to fears of returning to alcohol abuse. The patient was hospitalized in an anxious frenzy at a local medicosurgical hospital by her psychologist and a family practitioner. The two doctors proceeded to detoxify the patient, manage her overwhelming guilt and fears of impending doom, and avert a relapse to alcohol. After 4 days the patient was discharged without medications, with training in biofeedback and relaxation to manage anxiety, and was placed in aftercare with the addictions psychologist and the family physician. She was optimistic about her future, knew she had doctors whom she could rely on when rough spots in her recovery occurred, and had increased self-esteem based on mastery of an internally based skill for managing anxiety.

The psychologist working daily in the local rural outpatient delivery system will be the best prepared practitioner to effect referral and aftercare or to take on the commitment to follow the case post-hospitalization. The already burdened family physician in the rural area will have neither time nor training to provide or coordinate these substance abuse services. However, the family practice physician, the psychologist, and the hospital social worker can become a formidable collaborative practice team that is very attractive to third-party payers increasingly drawn to efficient outpatient interventions. The psychologist is the professional with the time, background, and expertise to evaluate the contribution of allied health professionals and to coordinate diagnostic, treatment, and placement services for addicted patients who typically present with a complex array of mental, familial, legal, social, vocational, and educational disorders.

Coordinating Services

The systemic lack of availability of psychologist diagnosticians screening for substance abuse and dependence has resulted in missed diagnosis and inappropriate and overuse of Alcoholics Anonymous and self-help approaches (Morris, 1993). Substance abuse and mental health services have become fragmented and dispersed outside the grass roots primary health care system. This fragmentation has resulted in political and turf battles, unnecessary duplication of services, poor coordination and collaboration, barriers to the patient's access to appropriate services, and removal of the influence of the family practice physician and hospital from the substance abuse delivery system. The pattern of fragmentation and lack of availability of specialized addictions services is especially apparent in the rural hospital. The collaboration among doctors of medicine, osteopathy, and psychology at the local rural hospital will effectively reverse this trend, integrating the treatment of the substance abuser with the hospital and primary care delivery system.

Integrating psychologists who have specialized substance abuse assessment and treatment backgrounds with the rural hospital professional staff significantly strengthens the rural health care system. First, rural communities with psychologists become better able to recruit doctors specializing in substance abuse because of increased diagnostic and treatment work availability. Second, rural hospitals can increase revenue and stabilize budgets by adding substance abuse patients and referral networks. Finally, multidisciplinary approaches create the image and realistic base of a comprehensive service.

As noted in earlier chapters, recent changes at the federal level, including modifications to the Social Security Act, have allowed physicians to transfer some or all of the responsibility and liability of care for behavioral and addiction problems in hospital settings to psychologists (Ludwigsen, 1992, 1993; Morris, 1993; Social Security Administration, 1993). These changes provide broadening opportunities for the family physician and psychologist to collaborate on substance abuse cases requiring a great deal of medical and psychological expertise.

Increasingly, rural family practice physicians and psychologists are collaborating to provide comprehensive health care services. It is estimated that the vast majority of illnesses treated by the family practitioner have psychosocial causes (Kroenke & Mangelsdorff, 1989). As noted in Table 1 only 33% of patients presenting with common symptoms were found by expensive medical testing to have organic etiology. Others have noted that as much as 50% of medical outpatient visits are for psychosocial reasons (Katon, Kleinman, & Rosen, 1982; Stosokla, Zola, & Davidson, 1984). In Kroenke and

Table 1

Diagnostic Evaluation of 14 Common Symptoms

Symptom	No. evaluated %		No. of organic diagnoses discovered by testing[a]	Estimated cost (dollars)	
				Per evaluation	Per organic diagnosis[a]
Chest pain	80	83	5	272	4,354
Fatigue	57	70	5	130	1,486
Dizziness	34	62	3	223	2,532
Headache	20	38	1	389	7,778
Edema	26	58	4	122	793
Back pain	31	76	1	234	7,263
Dyspnea	31	84	9	209	720
Insomnia	6	18	0	110	
Abdominal pain	27	90	3	202	1,816
Numbness	17	86	2	160	1,384
Impotence	13	54	2	161	1,046
Weight loss	18	100	0	325	
Cough	15	100	2	147	1,104
Constipation	7	18	0	409	
Total	382	67	37	218	2,252

Note: Empty cells indicate that data were indeterminate because no organic diagnoses were discovered by testing. Table from "Common Symptoms in Ambulatory Care: Incidence, Evaluation, Therapy and Outcome," by K. Kroenke and D. Mangelsdorff, 1989, *American Journal of Medicine, 86,* p. 264. Copyright 1989 by Excerpta Medica, Inc. Reprinted with permission.
[a] Includes only those diagnoses not apparent after initial interview and physical examination.

Mangelsdorff's (1989) study, many of the symptoms noted in patients who sought help at primary care centers and hospitals were pathognomonic for substance abuse problems: chest pain, dizziness, headache, insomnia, abdominal pain, numbness, impotence, weight loss, and cough.

Case History

Betty, a 54-year-old married woman, was presented in the hospital 24 hours after admission. She had curled herself into the fetal position, was electively mute, and refused to eat. An interview with Betty's physician and husband revealed that Betty had been repeatedly hospitalized for various medical problems, including severe spasmodic colon, chest pains with related gastrointestinal problems, and stomach ulcers, and she was wont to require frequent outpatient appointments for years for general malaise with low energy, flulike symptoms, and obvious unhappiness. She had been treated with various psychotropic medications by a number of doctors over the years ranging from antidepressants, minor tranquilizers, tylenol with codeine, to synthetic narcotics. The husband described his wife as childlike with few interests or friends, and preferring to stay at home. He indicated that she had always been afraid of people, wouldn't shop alone, and had never learned to drive. The husband, who had been diagnosed with terminal cancer, was hostile, controlling, and made it clear that he consciously overprotected his wife often firing doctors who wouldn't do as he directed with her. The internist seeing her had run every costly medical lab study, including every advanced coronary, pulmonary, central nervous system, and muscle study known, and had found no noteworthy biological anomaly. All of the many hospitalizations had been in a medicosurgical hospital. Finally, with her insurance carrier beginning to resist all outpatient and inpatient treatment, a psychologist with hospital privileges was asked to consult on the case.

The psychologist hypnotized the patient to bring her out of her mutism and motoric withdrawal. During the hypnosis she related her anger at her husband's impending death and concern that she would not be able to function alone. She moved rapidly from affective and ego states and was momentarily depressed, panicky, seductive, and coquettish. She was, as her husband had described, childlike. The psychologist suggested during hypnosis that she was no longer alone and that he would be with her through the death of her husband and the reconstruction of her life. He indicated that she could remain in her curled and mute position for the evening but that by morning she would return to a well-rested, social, and interactive state. As indicated by the psychologist Betty returned to a calm state the next morning.

The patient progressed nicely in psychotherapy and was able to manage the death of her husband several months hence. She rebuilt her life and social circles, mastered shopping and driving, and took over the husband's orchard, garden, and farm management. After 2 years of treatment Betty was without medications, excited about life, and could discuss openly the years of verbal abuse, rigidity, and cruelty from her husband, while maintaining her love for him and honoring his memory.

Betty has been without psychotherapy or medications for 5 years; she has not been hospitalized in 7 years. She rarely needs medical care, making her insurance carrier happier.

Betty is living proof that the best managed care is comprehensive and accurate diagnosis based on an early targeting of the most likely causes for a disorder and followed by appropriate treatment. Betty's mental health needs were neglected for years by an internist who either didn't recognize the mental illness and related family mental illness or who did not know what constitutes appropriate care. Betty, and her husband, lost what could have been many happier and more constructive years of her life. Betty knows this now but bears no one malice.

As the burden for substance abuse services in the rural area shifts to the rural hospital and integrated primary care centers with multidisciplinary staff, the opportunity for collaboration between psychologists and physicians will expand (Bray & Rogers, 1995).

Recommendations

The move to limit hospital cost overruns in the Medicaid system, to shift patients to outpatient and community living, and to gain access to care for chronic patients has created a

ballooning of the number of patients with chemical dependency and mental disorder who will be seen in the rural
hospital and primary care setting. This increase will result in
pressure to reintegrate the fragmented physical and mental
health and substance abuse delivery systems. The traditional
primary care center is not equipped to meet this demand for
a broad array of health care needs. As noted in a National
Academy of Sciences report (Mazade, 1990),

> The committee therefore believes that all persons coming
> for care to medical settings should be screened for alco-
> hol problems. If mild or moderate problems are present,
> a brief intervention should be provided in situation and
> observed for its effect. If substantial or severe substance
> abuse problems are present, a referral to specialized
> treatment should be initiated.

Unless the primary care setting is modified to include multidisciplinary staffing patterns, broad service delivery capacity, and psychological and chemical dependency leadership,
the deinstitutionalization movement will fail or result in a
repeat of the fragmentation of previous health care delivery
systems. The definition of primary health care must be broadened to encompass the treatment of substance abusers and
the mentally ill who are in the primary care population in
significant numbers.

The rural hospital has a unique opportunity to become the
guiding comprehensive force in the identification and treatment of patients with a primary or secondary diagnosis of
substance abuse or addiction. The psychologist can play an
important role in the delivery and management of these services in the hospital and in the outpatient service delivery
network. To accomplish this integration of physical and behavioral health and substance abuse services, the rural hospital will need to integrate psychologists into the medical–
professional staff and take advantage of federal and state rule
changes relative to the psychologist's scope of practice. Rural
hospitals that are able to do so will be in an advantageous
position.

References

APA Office of Rural Health. (1994). *Caring for the Rural Community: An Interdisciplinary Curriculum*. Washington, DC: American Psychological Association.

Baird, M. A., Burge, S. K., & Grant, W. D. (1989). A scheme for determining the prevalence of alcoholism in hospitalized patients. *Alcoholism: Clinical and Experimental Research, 13*, 782–785.

Baker, F., Jodrey, D., Intagliatia, J., & Straus, H. (1993). Community support services and functioning of the seriously mentally ill. *Community Mental Health Journal, 29*, 321–331.

Barker, P., Manderscheid, R., Hendershot, G., Jack, S., Schoenborn, C., & Goldstrom, I. (1989). *Serious mental disability in the adult household population: United States, 1989*. In R. Manderscheid & M. Sonnerschein (Eds.), Mental health, United States, 1992. Washington, DC: U.S. Government Printing Office.

Boydston, J. C. (1983). Rural mental health: A partnership with physicians. *Practice Digest, 6*, 23–25.

Bradley, K. A. (1992). Screening and diagnosis of alcoholism in the primary care setting. *Western Journal of Medicine, 156*, 166–171.

Bray, J. H., & Rogers, J. C. (1995). Linking psychologists and family physicians for collaborative practice. *Professional Psychology: Research and Practice, 26*, 132–138.

Broskowski, A. (1980). *Evaluation of the primary healthcare project-community mental health center initiative: Executive summary* (Contract No. 278-79-0030). Washington, DC: Department of Health and Human Services, Alcohol, Drug Abuse, and Mental Health Administration, National Institute of Mental Health.

Brown, R. L., Carter, W. B., & Gordon, M. J. (1987). Diagnosis of alcoholism in a simulated patient encounter by primary care physicians. *Journal of Family Practice, 25*, 259–264.

Buie, J. (1990, January). Rural therapists often advise MDs on drugs. *The APA Monitor, 21*, 19.

Burns, B. J., Burke, J. D., Jr., & Ozarin, L. D. (1983). Linking health and mental health services in rural areas. *International Journal of Mental Health, 12* (1–2), 130–143.

Candib, L., & Glenn, M. (1983). Family medicine and family therapy: Comparative development, methods, and roles. *Journal of Family Practice, 16*, 773–779.

Celenza, C. M., & Fenton, D. N. (1981). Integrating mental and medical health services: The Kennebec–Somerset Model. *New Directions for Mental Health Services, 9*, 39–49.

Chan, A. W. K., Pristach, E. A., & Welte, J. W. (1994). Detection by the

CAGE of alcoholism or heavy drinking in primary care outpatients and the general population. *Journal of Substance Abuse, 6,* 123–135.

Coulehan, J. L., Zettler-Segal, M., Block, M., McClelland, M., & Schulberg, H. C. (1987). Recognition of alcoholism and substance abuse in primary care patients. *Archives of Internal Medicine, 147,* 249–352.

Cummings, N. A., Dorkin, H., Pallak, M. S., & Henke, C. (1990). *The impact of psychological intervention on health care utilization and costs: The Hawaii Medicaid Project* (Report No. 11-C-98344/9). San Francisco: Biodyne Institute.

Cummings, N. A., & Follette, W. T. (1968). Psychiatric services and medical utilization in a prepaid health plan setting: Part II. *Medical Care, 6,* 31–41.

Durell, J., Lechtenberg, B., Corse, S., & Frances, R. (1993). Alcohol and drug abuse: Intensive case management of persons with chronic mental illness who abuse substances. *Hospital and Community Psychiatry, 44,* 415–416, 428.

Dym, B., & Berman, S. (1986). The primary health care team: Family physician and family therapist in joint practice. *Family Systems Medicine, 4,* 9–21.

Eichmann, M. A., Griffin, B. P., Lyons, J. S., Larson, D. B., & Finkel, S. (1992). An estimation of the impact of OBRA-877 on nursing home care in the United States. *Hospital and Community Psychiatry, 43,* 781.

Enright, M. F., & Blue, B. A. (1989). Collaborative treatment of panic disorders by psychologists and family physicians. *Psychotherapy in Private Practice, 7,* 85–90.

Follette, W. T., & Cummings, N. A. (1967). Psychiatric services and medical utilization in a prepaid health plan setting. *Medical Care, 5,* 25–35.

Graham, A. W. (1991). Screening for alcoholism by life-style risk assessment in a community hospital. *Archives of Internal Medicine, 151,* 958–964.

Hartman-Stein, P. E., & Reuter, J. M. (1993). *Proactive health care reform: Integrating physical and psychological care.* Unpublished paper.

Health Care Is Taking a Bigger Bite From Family Budgets; Businesses are Paying More, Too. (1993, March–April). *Health Beat: Rural Health News Update & Review,* p. 1.

Hiller, W., Mombour, W., & Mittlehammer, J. (1989). A systematic evaluation of the *DSM–III–R* criteria for alcohol dependence. *Comprehensive Psychiatry, 30,* 403–415.

Hoffman, A. L., & Slade, J. (1992). Following the pioneers: Addressing tobacco in chemical dependency treatment. *Journal of Substance Abuse Treatment, 10,* 153–160.

Janis, I. (1984). The patient as decision maker. In D. W. Gentry (Ed.), *Handbook of behavioral medicine.* New York: Guilford Press.

Jarman, C. M. B., & Kellet, J. M. (1979). Alcoholism in the general hospital. *British Medical Journal, 2,* 469–472.

Kaplan, H. I., & Sadock, B. J. (Eds.). (1985). *Comprehensive textbook of psychiatry/IV*. Baltimore: Williams & Wilkins.

Katon, W., Kleinman, A., & Rosen, G. (1982). Depression and somatization: A review. *American Journal of Medicine, 72*, 127–135, 241–247.

Koyanagi, C., Manes, J., Surles, R., & Goldman, H. H. (1993). On being very smart: The mental health community's response in the health care reform debate. *Hospital and Community Psychiatry, 44*, 537–542.

Krantz, D. S., & Glass, D. C. (1984). Personality, behavior patterns, & physical illness: Conceptual & methodological issues. In D. W. Gentry (Ed.), *Handbook of behavioral medicine* (pp. 38–86). New York: Guilford Press.

Kroenke, K., & Mangelsdorff, D. (1989). Common symptoms in ambulatory care: Incidence, evaluation, therapy, and outcome. *American Journal of Medicine, 86*, 262–266.

Leventhal, H., Zimmerman, R., & Gutman, M. (1984). Compliance: A self-regulation perspective. In D. W. Gentry (Ed.), *Handbook of behavioral medicine* (pp. 369–436). New York: Guilford Press.

Ludwigsen, K. R. (1992). Training psychologists for hospital practice. *Register Report, 18*, pp. 8, 14, 23–24.

Ludwigsen, K. R. (1993). Advocacy issues in hospital practice. *Independent Practitioner, 13*, 174–176.

Mazade, L. (Ed.). (1990). *Broadening the base of treatment for alcohol problems*. Washington, DC: National Academy Press.

McLellan, A. T., Arndt, I. O., Metzger, D. S., Woody, G. E., & O'Brien, C. P. (1993). The effects of psychosocial services in substance abuse treatment. *JAMA, 269*, 1953–1959.

Merline, J. (1993, May 26). The long term care time bomb. *Investor's Business Daily*, 1–2.

Moore, R. A. (1971). The prevalence of alcoholism in a community general hospital. *American Journal of Psychiatry, 128*, 130–131.

Moore, R. D., & Malitz, F. E. (1986). Underdiagnosis of alcoholism by residents in an ambulatory medical practice. *Journal of Medical Education, 61*, 46–52.

Morris, J. A. (1993). Health care trends: Hospital and healthcare facilities committee scores a victory. *The Independent Practitioner, 13*, 209–212.

Morris, J. A. (1994). The history of managed care and its impact on psychodynamic treatment. *Journal of Psychoanalysis and Psychotherapy, 11*, 129–137.

Morris, J. A., & Wise, R. P. (1992). The identification and treatment of the dual diagnosis patient. *Alcoholism Treatment Quarterly, 9*, 55–64.

Parker, D. A., & Harford, T. C. (1992). The epidemiology of alcohol consumption and dependence across occupations in the United States. *Alcohol Health & Research World, 16*, 97–105.

Regier, D. A., Farmer, M. E., Rae, D. S., Locke, B. Z., Keith, S. J., Judd, L. L., & Goodwin, F. K. (1990). Comorbidity of mental disorders with alcohol and other drug abuse results from the Epidemiologic Catchment Area (ECA) study. *JAMA, 264,* 2511–2518.

Reiger, D. A., Myers, J. K., Kramer, M., Robins, L. N., Blazer, D. G., Hough, R. L., Eaton, W. W., & Locke, B. Z. (1984). The NIMH Epidemiologic Catchment Area program: Historical context, major objectives, and study population characteristics. *Archives of General Psychiatry, 41,* 934–941.

Reid, A. L. A., Webb, G. R., Hennrikus, D., Fahey, P. P., & Sanson-Fisher, R. W. (1986). General practitioner's detection of patients with high alcohol intake. *British Medical Journal, 293,* 735–737.

Rice, D. P. (1993). The economic cost of alcohol abuse and alcohol dependence: 1990. *Alcohol Health & Research World, 17,* 10–11.

Schuckit, M. A. (1987). Why don't we diagnose alcoholism in our patients? *Journal of Family Practice, 25,* 225–226.

Social Security Administration. (1993). Sec. 1861(f), 42 U.S.C. 1395x. Compilation of the Social Security Laws (Committee Print WMCP: 103-5). Washington, DC: U.S. Government Printing Office.

Sperry, P. (1993, May 25). High tech medicine's high cost. *Investor's Business Daily,* pp. 1, 2.

Stosokla, J. D., Zola, I. K., & Davidson, G. E. (1984). The quantity and significance of psychological distress in medical patients. *Journal of Chronic Disorders, 17,* 969–970.

Umbrecht-Schneiter, A., Santora, P., & Moore, R. D. (1991). Alcohol abuse: Comparison of two methods for assessing its prevalence and associated morbidity in hospitalized patients. *American Journal of Medicine, 91,* 110–118.

VandenBos, G. (1993). U.S. mental health policy. Proactive evaluation in the midst of health care reform. *American Psychologist, 48,* 283–290.

White House Domestic Policy Council. (1993). *The president's health security plan* (1st ed.). New York: Random House.

Appendix

American Psychological Association Rural Health Task Force

Michael F. Enright, PhD, Chair
P.O. Box 4120
Medical Arts Building
557 East Broadway
Jackson, WY 83001-4120

James H. Bray, PhD
Department of Family Medicine
Baylor College of Medicine
5510 Greenbriar
Houston, TX 77005

Paul L. Craig, PhD
3260 Providence Drive, Suite 422
Anchorage, AK 99508-4615

David S. Hargrove, PhD
Department of Psychology
University of Mississippi
University, MS 38677

Mary Beth Kenkel, PhD
California School of Professional Psychology
1350 M Street
Fresno, CA 93721-1881

Arthur McDonald, PhD
Dull Knife Memorial College
P.O. Box 98
Lame Deer, MT 59043

Jerry A. Morris, PsyD
Community Mental Health Consultants, Inc.
815 South Ash
Nevada, MO 64772

Sylvia Shellenberger, PhD
3780 Eisenhower Parkway
Macon, GA 31206

Staff Liaison:
James G. Hill
American Psychological Association
Office of Rural Health Initiatives
Practice Directorate
750 First Street, NE
Washington, DC 20002-4242

Division of Independent Practice (42) Hospital and Health Care Facilities Committee

Jerry A. Morris, PsyD, Chair
Community Mental Health Consultants, Inc.
815 South Ash
Nevada, MO 64772

Jeannie Beeaff
Division of Independent Practice (42)
Central Office
919 Marshall Avenue
Phoenix, AZ 85013

Index

26–27. *See also* Collaborative
practice
Cost(s)
hospital and drugs vs. outpatient, 41
and Medicaid patients with substance abuse disorders, 129
of organic diagnosis, 136
Cost containment
and case management, 43–44
interventions effective in, 115
and managed care, 38, 42, 132
in Medicaid system, 138
Cost-effectiveness, and psychological interventions, 91–92, 128–
31
Cost-offset benefits, of behavioral
health care, 68, 129
Credentialing
APA policy on, 10–11
and clinical neuropsychologist,
105–6
psychologists in process of, 22–
23
Task Force on, 6
Dentists, community education
and prevention efforts of, 102
Depression, in women, 124
Diagnosis
of alcoholism, 130
and case history (Betty), 138
by psychologist, 10
of women's biopsychosocial
problems, 123–24
Diagnostic related groups (DRGs),
42
Drug abuse
prevalence of, 84
and smoking, 128
See also Substance abuse

Eating disorders, 123
Education in community
by dentists, 102

by neuropsychologist, 102–3
on women's health issues
seminars, 118–19
support groups, 119–22
Emergency room, psychologist–
physician collaboration in, 81,
82–83, 92–93
accountability and cost-effectiveness in, 91–92
in disposition and treatment,
90–91
and evaluation process, 86–90
immediate response needed for,
87
and psychologist's functions, 86
specific variables for, 83–86
Emotional factors, collaborative
practice impeded by, 59–60
Environmental changes, as neuropsychological treatment, 103
*Ethical Principles of Psychologists
and Code of Conduct* (APA),
25–26
Ethical standards or issues, 25–26
and ER calls, 87
as psychologist's consideration,
47–48

Family physicians, 58
psychologists in collaboration
with, 7
psychosocial causes confronted
by, 135
See also Primary care physicians
Family therapy, and managed-care
service, 43
Financial arrangements, and physicians vs. psychologists, 61
Financial incentives, xx
Freedom of choice laws, 23

*Guidelines on Hospital Privileges:
Credentialing and Bylaws*
(APA), 11

About the Editor

Jerry A. Morris, PsyD, is currently the clinical director and co-owner of Community Mental Health Consultants, Inc., a network of five comprehensive community mental health centers covering 27 counties in both rural and urban Missouri. He is a developer and former owner of a 47-bed psychiatric hospital.

Dr. Morris is a licensed clinical psychologist, a member of the International Council of Psychologists and APA Divisions 12, 22, 31, 40, 42, 43, and 50. He serves as the Division 42 chairperson of the Hospital and Healthcare Facilities Committee (1991–1997), has chaired the Division 43 Committee on Rural Family Psychology, and has served as the Division 42 National Grass Roots coordinator. Dr. Morris is also a member of the APA Interdivisional Committee on Health Care Reform, was a charter member of the APA Task Force on Rural Psychology, and is currently a member of the APA Rural Health Committee.

Dr. Morris has published and conducted research on the following topics: addiction, prevalence of co-morbidity or psychopathology of addicted persons, children and spouses of addicted persons, family therapy, multidisciplinary day treatment center approaches to the treatment of addiction, ethics, and hospital practice.